SAVING REBECCA

A Mother's Journey and Triumph into the Unexpected World of ADHD and Disability

Shirl Crimmins Smith

Saving Rebecca

A Mother's Journey and Triumph into the Unexpected World of ADHD and Disability
By Shirl Crimmins Smith

Copyright © 2019. Shirl Crimmins Smith. All rights reserved. No part of this publication may be reproduced, distributed, or transmitted in any form or by any means, including photocopying, recording, or other electronic or mechanical methods, without the prior written permission of the publisher, except in the case of brief quotations embodied in critical reviews and certain other noncommercial uses permitted by copyright law.

Publishing imprint Shirl\Crimmins Smith

ISBN: 978-0-578-57528-5

Please add this Disclaimer:

This book is not intended to be a substitute for the medical advice of a medical professional. The reader is advised to regularly consult with a physician in matters relating to his/her health or that of their child, and particularly concerning any symptoms that may require medical attention. I have tried to recreate events, locales, and conversations to the best of my ability from my memories. Although the author and publisher have made every effort to ensure that the information in this book was correct at press time, the author and publisher do not assume and hereby disclaim any liability to any party for any loss, damage, or disruption caused by errors or omissions, whether such errors or omissions result from negligence, accident, or any other cause.

Printed in the United States of America.

To Rebecca, who taught me so much on our life journey and showed, by example, how a person endures difficult struggles with dignity and determination. I am a better person and mom because of the adversity we endured to achieve our successes. You truly are an inspiration for others as to what a person can achieve in life when they have the fortitude and desire.

In loving memory of Shawn Michael Crimmins
March 2, 1975 – September 16, 2019

Also, in memory of my nephew Shawn, who left us suddenly and forever changed our lives. In my desperate need to find some solace for this devastation, I pulled out a card he had sent me many years ago where he shared these precious words.

Aunt Shirl,

Thank you for being the best Aunt anyone could ever wish for. Keep working on your book – I know you'll make it!

Love,
Shawn

Thank you, my sweet young Shawn, for always believing that I had the ability to create a book that could help others and change lives. Always and forever, in my heart.

Acknowledgments

There are too many people to thank individually for helping me learn how to adapt and raise a special needs child. So, to my family, friends, teachers, and other parents, a heartfelt thank you for your love and support. A very special thank you to my hubby Greg, for being my best friend and always supporting my latest discovery or whim. To Stephanie, my first born, I would not have accomplished what I did without your deep devotion to Rebecca, always watching my back, and being another set of eyes. Your support, wisdom, and compassion were truly a gift from God. A huge appreciation to my parents, siblings, and extended family for their unwavering belief that I could move mountains. To all the fantastic teachers who believed in Rebecca and helped her attain an education. Thank you. Finally, to the Four most remarkable women instrumental in Rebeccas success in life, Margo, Sheryl, Elizabeth, and Rita. Without your support and incredible devotion as teachers, Rebecca would never have accomplished the life she has today. God Bless you all.

Table of Contents

INTRODUCTION: How I Became Me ix

CHAPTER ONE: Early Morning Jitters 1

CHAPTER TWO: Rebecca's Journey 13

CHAPTER THREE: The Desperate Search for Knowledge 27

CHAPTER FOUR: The Man Behind the Diet 47

CHAPTER FIVE: Learning to Use the Feingold Diet 59

CHAPTER SIX: The Launching of Kindergarten 73

CHAPTER SEVEN: The Fork in the Road 89

CHAPTER EIGHT: Maneuvering the School Years 107

CHAPTER NINE: Life After High School 125

CHAPTER TEN: Looking Back at Our Love Story 141

Introduction

Have you ever wanted to vanish the moment your child became a screaming mess in public and all eyes turned to you as though you were the worst parent on the planet? Do you dread every outing and pray this time your child will not create a scene? If so, I bet you have wondered what the heck happened to that precious little bundle of joy you brought home two or three years ago. No, I am not one of those condemning people, nor have I peeked in your window. I am one of those parents who had an unruly child who was extremely physical and raged and screamed like a banshee. What if I told you that I was asked to remove my ADHD daughter from preschool and shortly after placing her in a specialized school she was on the verge of expulsion? It took this overwhelming situation and pressure to use medication that compelled me to search for a safe resolution for my daughter.

In about three weeks, she went from acting like the Tasmanian devil to a calm, happy, and more compliant child who just happened to have ADHD. This astounding outcome required my unwavering commitment to using consistent behavioral management strategies and removing all artificial ingredients from her food and drinks. *Saving Rebecca: A Mother's Journey and Triumph into the Unexpected World of ADHD and Disability,* you get a front-row seat to see how I conquered denial, overcame the struggles, healed emotional pain, and turned self-doubt into success.

Using expert help and self-education, I put the puzzle pieces together and created an effective plan of action that transformed our out-of-control daughter into a compliant child at home and school, despite having learning disabilities. I do acknowledge that in some cases medication may be the only option, but why not try three weeks of a safe alternative first? Parenthood is challenging enough without the complications of ADHD, let alone the side effects of the pharmaceuticals prescribed to manage it. In the U.S. alone, 6.4 million children aged four to seven have been diagnosed with ADHD, and it is time for their caregivers to seek out and demand other solutions, rather than relying on one that enriches drug companies while families suffer.

CHAPTER ONE

Early Morning Jitters

"Use what talents you possess; the woods would be very silent if no birds sang there except those that sang best."

Henry Van Dyke

The bedroom was still shadowed in darkness when at five-thirty a.m. the alarm roused us. As I lumbered about, preparing for our journey to the hospital, I couldn't shake the nagging feeling that even several hours of sleep had done little to quell. It was the feeling that something was wrong with the baby. I tried to convince myself that it was anxiousness about it being Friday the Thirteenth, and my belief that I was carrying a girl. When our first child, little Miss Stephanie, was born, my husband Greg had assured me that he was not disappointed, that the most important thing was that she was healthy. In his mind, little girls could learn to ride motorcycles too, and he was looking forward to sharing his passion with her. My apprehension, however, was that his reaction would not be the same when our second child also turned out to be a girl.

Since childhood I have always paid close attention to my intuition. Some think this is abnormal; indeed, if this heightened sixth sense was not also shared by some of my siblings I, too, would have seriously questioned my sanity. More often than not, these sensations have been confirmed, which has merely validated my belief that I was born this way. No doubt some of you may be rolling your eyes or thinking that superstitions are ridiculous, but for me, it was a constant component of my childhood. I watched adults whom I loved, respected, and adored become genuinely alarmed by certain situations or beliefs. Even my Grandma Crimmins, a devout Irish Catholic, did not leave her house until she checked her horoscope. When you grow up in that type of environment it seems perfectly reasonable to accept those beliefs, behaviors, and traditions. I guess you could say old habits die hard, if at all. Needless to say, when I woke up that morning still feeling apprehensive, I was on high alert mode.

As Greg headed downstairs to make coffee, I finished getting dressed, grabbed my suitcase, and went down to join him. Just walking into the kitchen made my stomach grumble in protest of the doctor's order of no food or drink before delivery. My natural tendency is to wake up ravenous and head straight for the cereal box to appease the beast. I also tend to get fixated on whatever I am being denied, and at that moment, it was food. Thankfully, I had yet to become a coffee drinker and waited to embrace that addiction until I was almost forty years old. Believe me when I say that my compulsive and fixated characteristic traits continue to bring both satisfaction and trouble into my life!

Greg suited up for his brisk encounter with the Iowa winter morning, then headed out to the garage in the back of the house; he would warm up the truck and pull around front to retrieve me. As I watched him trudge through the freshly fallen snow it occurred to me that the steps he took was not just a physical action, but also an integral part of life. Time is always moving us forward and propelling us to keep placing one foot in front of the other, regardless of our desires, circumstances and reservations. On that morning, my major reservation was the persistent foreboding and heaviness about my impending delivery. I cannot remember a time when my premonitions, dreams, or extreme sensitivities did not convey a sense of looming trouble or impending tragedy. These feelings were exacerbated by the fact that the forewarnings, though relentless, failed to reveal exact knowledge of what was approaching or who would be impacted. Before this impending alarm for the baby, there was only one time that I had had a sensation of imminent death, and we lost Merlyn, Greg's dad, the following day.

When I stepped outside, I was in utter amazement of the spectacular sight in the faint light of dawn. Not a trace of animal or human had marred the perfection of the snow that covered the lawns, street, and rooftops. Smoke drifted from the chimneys of the houses across the street, and the snow glistened like scattered diamonds beneath the streetlights. It was a magical sight to behold as I stood on the front steps in the brisk stillness of the frosty morning. This extraordinary picture of perfection seemed like a gift from God and created a comforting sense of tranquility that softly embraced me and quieted my apprehension. As I took in the beautiful vision, the silence was broken by the sound of Greg's truck coming around the corner and heading up the street. The sidewalks had yet to be shoveled, so I waited for him to help me down the front steps; then, with a firm hold on my arm he shadowed my footsteps until I was safely perched inside the truck. As silly as it sounds, my heart melted over that simple act of chivalry from my man of few words. It made me feel protected, cherished, and deeply loved.

Once we arrived at the hospital, I was taken to the maternity ward while Greg stayed behind to fill out the paperwork. After the nurse got me settled in bed, she inserted the IV drip into my hand to induce labor and then began the procedure of rupturing the bag of amniotic fluid. It was at this moment that poor Greg walked into the room and instantly stopped like a deer in the headlights. He was too far into the room to turn and run without being obvious, and so had to endure the extreme discomfort of witnessing the procedure. And then, at sixty-thirty a.m., the waiting began.

Rarely do things go smoothly where I am concerned, and that day was no different. When my contractions failed to accelerate as expected, the nurse speculated that the baby was resting too far out from the birth canal and left to consult with my doctor. His solution was to have her encase my stomach with an elastic girdle, so she brought an additional nurse to help with this process. This endeavor was comical, and I wished that I had had the forethought to bring a video-recorder because I would have won America's Funniest Videos! After a great deal of wrestling and heavy panting, they finally concurred that a larger size was necessary. After round two, these professionals succeeded in binding my massive baby mound and stood back grinning with great satisfaction. They were confident that this device would now apply enough pressure to push the baby back toward the birth canal and expedite my delivery.

Imagine everyone's surprise when nothing happened within the first hour, or even after the second, even as the contractions relentlessly assaulted my body. I watched enviously as the woman from the room next to mine was wheeled past the doorway toward the delivery room. She was followed a short time later by another gurney, this time with a woman who had come to the floor after my arrival. It seemed cruel and unfair that they advanced to the finish line while I was stuck in this limbo of pain. In my frustrated state, a vivid picture of Whales popped into my mind. No doubt, this thought was provoked by being confined to bed while the girdle was forcefully squeezing my belly. It made me contemplate if this was how a beached whale felt as it watched its species swim away while it remained trapped on shore.

After six grueling hours, the contractions were coming so quickly that I could no longer regulate my breathing or prepare for the next one before it ripped through my body. Greg watched helplessly while I struggled and grew increasingly exhausted, irritable, and queasy. As the pain became intolerable, I growled at him to run a paper towel under cold water and bring it over to me. He was noticeably hesitant to walk over to the bed and within proximity of my agitated state. His concern was not unfounded, as at that miserable moment I was not above violence. What woman does not have such feelings during childbirth? My mom often warned me about my facial expressions being a window to my thoughts, and apparently, my face was revealing signs of hostility toward Greg.

Greg had been spared from watching this struggle four years earlier when I gave birth to Stephanie. That time I had followed my mom's advice and walked through my contractions. Mom, who had given birth to nine children, told me this would make natural childbirth easier. With my sister Cindy as my walking companion and timekeeper, I wandered the streets of our childhood neighborhood for hours until the contractions reached the three-minute interval. At that point, she took me home to wake up Greg so that he could take me to the hospital. As it turned out, Mom was right; I had delivered within three hours of arriving at the hospital!

Greg advanced toward the bed and timidly held out the towel, which I snatched ungraciously from his hand and snapped "thank you"; then he quickly retreated to the chair in the corner. My ugly side tends to surface when I am in excessive pain, making me snap and snarl like a rabid dog. The cold towel refreshed my sweaty face and helped reduce nausea, and I sheepishly glanced over at Greg who was now quietly watching television. He must have felt my stare because he turned and looked at me with such genuine misery that it hit me how distressing it was for him watching me endure the pain of labor. I too would have hated watching him suffer and being unable to do a darn thing to help, and this reality check softened my less-than-charming disposition until the next contraction ripped through my body.

Attempting to breathe through the agony sent me deep within the confines of my memory. A scary place on a good day, but I was seeking insight as to why this birthing ritual was torturing me so when all I wanted was the misery to end and hold a healthy baby in my arms. The only insight that came to mind was that life invariably gives everyone challenges and blessings, and for whatever reason, this challenge was somehow supposed to enrich my life.

I couldn't help but reflect upon one blessing in particular, the one who had ridden into my life, not as a knight in shining armor, but a tall, handsome man astride his motorcycle. My younger brother Tom had met Greg while they rode their dirt bikes on the trails outside of town on the weekends. Greg and I were in the same high school graduating class of 1974, though our paths never crossed during those three years. It was through sharing stories that we came to realize that Greg was the anonymous person who had been instrumental in saving Tom's life many years before. While swimming at the YMCA, he had been knocked unconscious and Greg's quick alarm enabled the lifeguards to resuscitate Tom while waiting for the ambulance. Thankfully, my brother suffered no permanent brain damage and was home the next day.

Tom was convinced that Greg was the perfect man for me and insisted on introducing us. At the time, my social life had been more pain than joy, so I was extremely resistant to the meet and greet. Tom, being the more stubborn sibling, refused to accept my excuses and I finally agreed, more to get him off my back than out of any genuine interest. Tom arranged for a meeting at the movie theater where he worked, and I enlisted our sister Pat, the sibling between us, to be my moral support. That day, Pat and I arrived beforehand to watch the movie, and once the theatre was empty, Greg came. Tom made the introductions, and it turned out Greg was no better at small talk than I was. After a polite but awkward exchange, he walked away and went outside.

As I watched his retreating figure I was left with the feeling that this had been a total waste of time and I should have held firm to my conviction rather than caving to Tom's wishes. I had just grabbed my purse to leave when I heard the rumbling of a motorcycle. I turned to see Greg come riding through the entrance of the theatre. He rode past the three of us and into the seating area, down one aisle, across the front, and then back up the other aisle. With a satisfied grin on his face, he rode past us and out the front door! For one shocked moment my siblings and I stood there like the three stooges, then Tom let out a sidesplitting laugh. When we looked outside we saw that Greg had just pulled his motorcycle up into a wheelie and was riding away. I turned to Tom, confused and disappointed that he thought introducing me to this crazy dude was a good fit for my commonsense mentality.

Tom and Pat, on the other hand, thought Greg's antics were hilarious, though it was the intense shock on my face that gave Tom the most pleasure. When he asked what I thought of Greg, my instant response was that it might be a good thing if I never saw him again. This was all Pat needed to hear. Without hesitation, my thrill-seeking sister proclaimed that whomever Greg asked out would get him, then she thrust out her hand for me to shake in agreement. As if the two of us had any ownership of this stranger our adoring brother called a friend.

Several weeks later Pat and I were leaving to get something to eat when Tom and Greg rode up on their motorcycles. Just being polite, I asked if they wanted me to bring something back for them and they requested cheeseburgers. As we drove to McDonald's, I made it clear to Pat that when we returned it would be only to drop off the food and leave because I was not eager to have another interaction with Greg. Though my dating experience was not extensive, I knew that Greg was different from the few guys that I had dated. He radiated a strong masculinity that scared me a wee little bit, an emotion I had not experienced before. I also felt he was entirely out of my league. My life was finally uncomplicated from trying to make past relationships work, and I had no desire to relinquish my liberation by contemplating the distraction of dating again.

Fate, however, was insistent upon our paths crossing again. While leaving work for lunch, I ran into Greg who had been sent to Safeway to perform a plumbing service call. He thanked me for buying him the cheeseburger and asked me out to dinner, he said to repay my kindness. Before I knew it I found myself agreeing to dinner with him that weekend, then chewing out my own ass as I walked away. Damned if I had not let his dashing good looks and enticing smile dissolve my instinct to stay away from him.

I spent the rest of the week stressing about the date, only to be surprised again, this time pleasantly so, when the evening turned out to be relaxed and quite enjoyable. Greg was mature, charming and entertaining – a vast improvement from my prior experiences. He also was (and still is) a handsome devil with an adorable grin that highlighted and complimented his quick wit.

That date was only the beginning, and as we spent more time together, I got to know the man behind the smile. I found him to be an honorable man who shared the same life values, and for the first time, I considered the possibility that he might be the man of my dreams. And, the rest, as they say, is history.

An intense contraction slammed me back into the present, accompanied by an urge to scream or strike out at something. The nurse came to check on my progress, and Greg surprised me by insisting that she ask my doctor for something to manage the pain. Unfortunately, this left my sweet hubby alone with me just as another contraction hit. A second later, he found himself struck in the face by the wet paper towel I had hurled across the room with surprising accuracy. I fully expected him to yell, "What the hell?" but he just flashed his famous grin and asked if that meant I wanted him to run it under cold water again. His self-control and sense of humor was my undoing, and I blurted out that the baby was going to be a girl and I could not remember how to spell the name we chose. He sat there for a moment staring at me and then, without a word, stood up and walked out.

As I heard his footsteps in the hall, I tried to ease my conscience by telling myself it's hard to be nice when another human being is attempting to rip open your stomach from the inside out. Even in my agony, I couldn't help but compare this experience to the relative ease of Stephanie's birth. Having the labor induced had created a constant bombardment of contractions with only brief moments in between to catch my breath. My pain tolerance was virtually nonexistent by this time, and as is my character, I had lashed out. The shame and guilt I felt for my inexcusable behavior assaulted my mind just as steadily as the pain of labor attacked my body.

My ability to withstand stressful situations has always depended dramatically on my mindset that I can handle just about anything.

Unfortunately, when I feel defenseless or vulnerable I lose control of my emotions, usually to the detriment of myself and anyone nearby. When I was growing up, it was impressed upon me that being born a Crimmins, and having an Irish pedigree, meant that I should not show fear or weakness. It was okay to have those emotions, but not to allow anyone to see them and therefore consider me weak. Right, wrong, or indifferent, that was the measuring stick of what it meant to have character, so to adapt to those expectations I created a mask to hide behind. Unfortunately, the pain of labor had caused my mask to slip.

When Greg walked out without saying a word, I believed he was trying to deal with the disappointment of not having a son, and the fact that I had failed him. A short while later he walked in, handed me a pamphlet of baby names, and replied, "Here is how we spell Rebecca." My sweet hubby had not left because he was upset but simply to find something with baby names. I know it sounds cliché, but I had honestly never loved him so deeply as I did at that moment. His thoughtfulness and insight were comforting, and just as I was starting to apologize, the nurse returned to perform another exam. What she discovered was the second bag of amniotic fluid that had been inhibiting my delivery. She suspected that the second bag was most likely due to me being pregnant with twins at the beginning of the pregnancy. Her statement confirmed my suspicions that I had suffered a miscarriage the day of Merlyn's funeral.

When Merlyn was killed by a drunk driver, I believed that I was pregnant but had yet to have it confirmed by my doctor. The senselessness of his death devastated our family as we grieved the loss of a devoted and loving son, brother, husband, father, and grandfather. The afternoon of his funeral, I experienced severe abdominal pain unlike anything I experienced before and assumed I had miscarried. My doctor had me come in for a blood test and called to tell me I was still pregnant; however, the cramping that I was feeling was my body fighting the pregnancy, and I was at high risk to suffer a miscarriage. I was closely monitored throughout my pregnancy, praying valiantly that our baby would keep fighting against the grieving process that was endangering its life.

The rupture of the second bag instantly revved up the process and within minutes I was being rushed to the delivery room. On the way out the door, the IV still attached to my hand became entangled on the door handle and abruptly halted my exit. The nurses worked frantically to get me free and wheeled me into the delivery room just as my doctor finished putting on his gown. He stepped over to the foot of the gurney for this long-awaited delivery, and Rebecca literally came shooting into the world. Her rapid delivery prevented anyone from knowing that the umbilical cord had wrapped around her neck and was strangling her.

Instantly my doctor began resuscitation efforts while I listened to his chant, "Come on baby, breathe, come on baby breathe." There was absolute silence except for his voice as everyone watched and waited for the sound of her victorious cry. Where was the spiritual high I felt as Stephanie came into the world head, shoulders, and body? She had made loud squawks of protest while the nurse cleaned her little pink body as she waved those long arms and legs as though trying to get somewhere.

The pandemonium of trying to revive Rebecca seemed to give more credence to my superstition about Friday the Thirteenth. Overwhelming terror consumed me as the sights, sounds, and smells were forever imprinted upon my mind. I prayed desperately to God for intervention, as we often do in times of a crisis, and promised to accept whatever complications came with Rebecca's traumatic birth if her life were spared. As I prayed, I sensed that Merlyn was present and helping his granddaughter from heaven and was instantly calmed as the second attempt at CPR successfully revived Rebecca. She was still not making a sound, and my doctor reassured me she was alive and breathing, but his attempt at smiling did not hide the look of concern on his face.

He handed Rebecca to the team and began tending to my medical needs, and I glanced over at her and saw the blue discoloring around her mouth, hands, and feet. She was cleaned, weighed, and measured, and then they gave me a quick glimpse before rushing her off to the nursery to be placed in an incubator. Greg's unease about coming into the delivery room had spared him the horror of witnessing what I had experienced and gratefully shielded him from the reoccurring nightmares that would torment me for years. Rebecca was born January 13, 1984, at 1:08 p.m. and even though the memory of her birth is forever imprinted on my mind, I no longer feel apprehension regarding Friday the Thirteenth. Because it was on that terrifying day that the Lord truly blessed our family with a miracle.

Rebecca was not the only baby to be born with the umbilical cord wrapped around her neck; in fact, it seemed to be a rather common occurrence in my family. It has, as far as I know, started with my brother Jim, followed by his son Joshua. Stephanie, my first child, also had the cord wrapped around her neck, but the delivery had been slow enough to allow sufficient time for it to be removed before she was in any real danger. After nearly losing Rebecca, I was determined to find out why this was happening, especially since there had been no indication of this life-threatening situation during either of my pregnancies. I spoke to several physicians and found that their data on this was vague. The only common thread with these types of births was that the mothers reported excessive activity during pregnancy. I was definitely more active with Rebecca than with Stephanie, however, since they had both been born with the cord wrapped around their necks this information, while insightful, did not prove anything.

Later, I would wonder if being born a "cord baby" had some connection with hyperactivity, but my research did not yield enough scientific evidence to either dispel or prove the theory. Still, Rebecca's rapid entrance into the world seemed to set a precedence for her life. Although she appeared to recover quickly from her traumatic birth, she showed difficulty catching her breath the following day as I attempted to feed her. I was not overly alarmed by this, as I had been born with asthma and my mom told me that I had done the same thing, but I did inform my doctor of the episode. Considering the circumstances under which she was born, my doctor ordered chest x-rays just to be on the safe side. The tests showed no abnormalities and we were released from the hospital three days later.

Several weeks later, Rebecca started vomiting after her feedings, and my doctor assumed it was most likely due to excess mucus remaining in her lungs from birth. Again, nothing for me to worry about. When I took her for her six-week check-up, the vomiting had yet to subside, but when I expressed my concern the doctor reminded me that Stephanie had also spit up after her feedings and outgrew the issue. He felt confident that it would be the same for Rebecca, and although his belief should have comforted me, the noticeable difference between the girls' symptoms bothered me. With Stephanie, it was more like "spit up," and with Rebecca, it was more like regurgitation. The persistent premonition that something was just not right would not stop churning in my gut.

CHAPTER TWO

Rebecca's Journey

"Start by doing what is necessary; then do what is possible, and suddenly you are doing the impossible."

St. Francis of Assisi

When Rebecca failed to gain weight and the vomiting persisted, my doctor felt it was time to run tests on her esophagus and stomach to rule out tumors, defects, and blockages. Thankfully, no abnormalities were discovered, and he believed the vomiting was the result of her traumatic birth. Since she tended to become overexcited at feeding time and gulped the formula rather than sucking it slowly, he prescribed medication to calm her before feedings. The hope was that she would be less inclined to guzzle and this would reduce the vomiting or eliminate it altogether. Unfortunately, it relaxed her throat too much. Formula came shooting out her nose and she started choking. At this point my doctor admitted he was at a loss and referred us to a specialist.

The pediatrician did suspect that Rebecca had a milk allergy, so he instructed me to discontinue the medication and substitute soymilk for the formula. Eliminating the drug stopped the choking, however, the soymilk had no effect on the vomiting. By this time I was really starting to fear for my daughter's life, and I said as much at our next appointment. The doctor stared at me for a moment, agreed she was in danger, and then declared that he believed her condition was due to me being either a neurotic mother or an incompetent one! For a moment, I sat there, so stunned and nauseated I had to fight being sick right there in front of him. Then, holding Rebecca more protectively to my chest, I just bolted out of his office.

As I marched down the hallway, the shock was replaced by anger, not only that he believed such things but had voiced them. It had been a long time since someone had rendered me speechless and unable to defend myself. I was neither neurotic nor incompetent; I was a mother who was desperate to save her child from starvation and had incurred substantial medical expenses trying to get answers that remained elusive to the medical professionals. As Rebecca's health continued to deteriorate, I could not find one physician who was able to determine a specific diagnosis or cure to the vomiting.

None of them knew about the link between vomiting after feedings and hyperactivity in infants. Indeed, no one even mentioned the possibility of hyperactivity, even though Dr. Ben Feingold's book *Why Your Child Is Hyperactive: The Bestselling Book on How ADHD is Caused by Artificial Food Flavors and Colors* had been published by Random House ten years earlier. My doctor did, however, contend that her problem was stress-related, which was not far off as anxiety is also a symptom of hyperactivity. To his credit, he also promptly referred me to a pediatric specialist when he was unable to diagnose Rebecca's ongoing health problems.

Four-year-old Stephanie seemed extraordinarily perceptive with regard to Rebecca's vulnerability and instinctively became her protector, which she still is today. I was proud of and amazed by Stephanie's ability to understand the circumstances surrounding her sister's struggles, as well as the depth of her compassion. Stephanie never appeared to harbor any resentment, jealousy, or animosity toward Rebecca for all the attention her sister required. It would have been normal for her to feel slighted after being the center of our world for four years and then have a sibling get so much attention. I was constantly in awe of my oldest child's ability to be that profoundly intuitive at such a young age.

In the coming months, we continued to struggle with Rebecca's persistent health problems. Despite our growing frustration with the professionals' lack of success, we believed we had no other recourse than to trust them. This was the mid-eighties, long before the age of Google, and information was much less readily available. Greg and I listened to their educated guesses and trial and error solutions, that is, until the day one of those specialists judged me an unfit mother! That was the breaking point for me, and it ticked me off enough to make me take matters into my own hands. After some research, I purchased a baby feeder typically used to help a child adapt to strained foods; this became Rebecca's bottle. Since she vomited the formula anyway, I replaced it with whole milk and added baby cereal to thicken the consistency. This method slowed down Rebecca's ability to power through her feedings and decreased the vomiting.

She was less frantic at her feedings and began to gain weight in pounds rather than ounces. Her pale complexion became healthy-looking, and her long arms and legs started to fill out, so now when we looked at her we no longer just saw a stomach protruding from malnutrition. Rebecca was finally thriving, which diminished my fear of her dying and ended my sleepless nights. When my primary doctor saw Rebecca at her scheduled check-up, he was pleased by her progress and assumed the pediatrician had successfully found an answer. I wasted no time enlightening him about my upset with that specialist and his inability to diagnose or cure the vomiting. When I shared how I had managed the improvement, he congratulated me on my ingenuity, which further validated my methods and it boosted my confidence. We both assumed things were finally on track, and Rebecca's struggles were now in the past.

Though Rebecca continued to gain weight, she also began to display changes in her behavior. She had never particularly liked being cuddled, but now she started struggling to be put down. There was also an increase in agitation and crying spells when she was in situations with high levels of noise or confusion, and the only way to calm her was by removing her to a quiet space. Even her sleep patterns changed, and she went from being a sound sleeper to a very light sleeper. Mom suggested playing a radio in her bedroom, which served as an effective sound barrier that helped her to fall asleep and stay asleep. Yet the behavioral changes continued with alarming regularity; in fact, the best way to describe this phenomenon was that each night I would put Rebecca to bed, only to find the next morning that she had yet another new quirk to her personality.

In the meantime, Stephanie had reached an exciting milestone: it was time for her to start preschool. She was a perpetually happy, loving, and extremely compassionate little girl, and I never doubted that she would adapt well to this new environment. Rebecca, however, had a tough time adjusting to Stephanie being gone and only perked up when it was time to get her from school. Yet, all in all, life finally seemed to be getting back on track - Stephanie was doing well in school and Rebecca was adapting to the new food choices I had introduced. I embraced the tranquility that comes from having a healthy, happy, and contented family. Then, just when I started to get comfortable, life thumped me upside the head with a substantial dose of reality. My illusion of harmony began to fracture as Rebecca started displaying more perplexing behaviors.

Whereas Stephanie was calm, happy, patient, and generally well behaved, Rebecca was extremely active, cranky, impatient and increasingly unruly. Clearly, the parenting skills that had been successful with one daughter was not going to work with the other. For example, Stephanie would instantly acknowledge my reprimands and stop whatever inappropriate behavior she happened to be engaged in; Rebecca would ignore me until I had to take further action (such as taking away an object she wasn't supposed to be playing with), then emit a howl of outrage like an angry bear. I was confused and frustrated by her unpredictable and aggressive behavior; I also believed that it was somehow my fault. Who else was there to blame? I was my children's primary caregiver.

Rebecca's aggression was just one of the things that concerned me. She also showed a delay in her speech development, so I asked my doctor to take a closer look. He could not find any medical signs to warrant my unease and believed the delayed speech was most likely due to her medical issues as an infant. As much as I wanted to embrace his assessment, my sixth sense had already sent up an alarm that something else was awry. To assuage my concerns, I went to the library to obtain a clear definition of child development. This venture was supposed to dispel my fears; instead, it validated my suspicions that Rebecca was behind in the developmental stages. Her temperament and speech patterns were not typical for a fourteen-month-old and no reassurance from my doctor, family or friends could dismiss my conviction that life was going to be difficult for Rebecca. That said, it was impossible to anticipate how complex the struggles would be or that they were behavioral problems distinct to hyperactivity.

To look at Rebecca, you saw this cute little girl with unruly blonde hair and beautiful sky-blue eyes that she had inherited from Grandpa Merlyn. She was a whirlwind of energy and an absolute charmer who had perfected her daddy's devilish grin. Rebecca was as entertaining as she was exasperating, and if her captive audience found her antics amusing, it only encouraged her escapades. I desperately wanted to embrace the notion that she was merely a spirited child, but the vivid memory of her birth lurked in the shadows of my mind with ominous warnings that there were deeper problems.

Our concern over the vocabulary delay soon became secondary to her drastic mood swings and latest inclination to bite without provocation. She only spoke one or two words to express herself, and if we failed to understand she resorted to pointing or taking us by the hand to what she desired. Since she was able to communicate her needs using this method, it was easier for us to believe that one day her speech limitations would improve. We were much more alarmed by her unlimited, frenetic energy that kept her in constant motion. It seemed she was always rocking, swaying, kicking and bouncing; in sleep, she tossed and turned so much that her legs would protrude outside the bars of her crib. I would be awakened to a horrifying scream and race to her room, automatically talking soothingly to avoid startling her before gently rubbing her legs. Once she was relaxed, I could bend her knees and get her legs back inside the crib. These episodes started becoming a weekly event, so we made the scary decision to take her out of the crib and put her in a twin bed. Greg stuffed pillows between the mattress and box spring on the outside edge so she would roll toward the wall and not fall out of bed.

Then there were the times when she would sit quietly on the floor and stare off into space. It was as though she had escaped into this hidden sanctuary inside her mind that only she could enter or understand. Sometimes I truly envied her that ability to retreat so profoundly within herself and appear peaceful. My life had become increasingly hectic and stressful, and it would have been heavenly to have a few minutes of that precious reprieve. The way that she could go from extreme movement to such total withdrawal cracked the protective cover of my denial. No longer did I believe that she would outgrow these behaviors, and it opened me up to the reality that Rebecca had developmental and behavioral issues. Looking for support, I shared my perceptions with family and friends who still believed she was just a spirited child, and I was a "worry wart." It seemed as if I was the only person to see a storm brewing, and my only uncertainty was just how battered our lives would be by it.

Unless Rebecca was sick, she woke up every morning energized and with one destination in mind, the quickest route to her highchair and breakfast. She would ravenously devour her meal with little regard to manners - something I attributed to her constant fight during infancy to survive - then follow up with a valiant attempt to outmaneuver the damp washcloth. As soon as she heard the click of the tray release on her chair, she was down and on the move. My non-stop performer of daredevil acts was determined to climb on, under, over, and between things all day long. Seven days a week, I endured a physical and mental work out as I tried to keep pace, restrain her fearlessness, and attempt to maintain some form of discipline.

Most often Rebecca interpreted the word NO as a challenge, which meant I was constantly removing her from kitchen counters, the stove, the kitchen table and the top of the refrigerator, and removing breakable items from her clutches. Many times, she retaliated by screaming, kicking, hitting, biting or pulling hair. A quick swat to her behind only provoked her anger and prolonged the temper tantrum. We encountered these battles of will repeatedly throughout the day, with her naptime our only ceasefire. While she slept and recharged her battery, I mentally tried to prepare for the next round, and bedtime never arrived soon enough! The only blessing from this madness was that it helped keep my weight down.

I called this stage of development the "terrifying twos syndrome of chaos." One minute, Rebecca would be playing contentedly and engrossed in an activity, and the next minute she'd be in the throes of a full-on tantrum. The source of her aggravation might be a block that had dared to tumble off the pile, a toy that refused to remain upright, or a person who had touched her toy. Since her moods fluctuated from contentment to fury with little to no warning, I always tried to be vigilant in monitoring her. I knew firsthand what she was physically capable of inflicting during a fit of anger and wanted to prevent that from happening to anyone else. Because of her high level of energy and aggressive nature, only Mom and a few siblings could endure the challenge of watching her while I ran errands.

One day, while Rebecca was playing with her toys, I told her to get her coat so that we could pick Stephanie up from preschool. When she ignored me, I assumed that she was being stubborn as usual and walked over and picked her up off the floor. Rebecca expelled this bone-chilling scream and started hitting me as I attempted to restrain her hands. It was at that moment, when I saw the pure terror on her face, that I realized she was not being defiant, she had not heard me talking to her. Instantly, my dad, who had suffered from an incurable inner ear bone disease, came to mind. Throughout my life his hearing had diminished, and when I was sixteen the FDA recalled the experimental drug that had stopped the progression of damage. Without that medication, the disease steadily worsened and he eventually became deaf. Fearing that Rebecca had inherited this disease, I immediately began searching for a facility to schedule a hearing test.

The audiologist at the Arrowhead Education Agency (AEA) found a substantial hearing loss in both ears and attributed it to ear infections. This confused me, because Rebecca, who had been plagued with ear infections from infancy, had not been exhibiting signs of them at the time. I made an appointment with an ear specialist who surgically inserted tubes in both ears, and Rebecca's hearing returned to normal. The tubes were expected to remain inside the inner ears for one year before gradually falling out, which it exactly what happened. Unfortunately, within a few days the fluid began building again, which necessitated another set of tubes. Here still, was another trait of hyperactivity, repeated episodes of ear infection in infants. Although the second set of tubes corrected the problem, the two surgeries resulted in moderate scarring of her inner ear.

Rebecca became more vocal after the ear surgeries and would proudly count to ten or sing her ABCs for anyone who would listen. Although her vocabulary increased, there was still a noticeable delay in her speech. The difficulty was not in her pronunciation of words, but more in choosing the correct words to give clarity to her sentences. Rebecca left out words or used unrelated words that made it difficult for her to communicate clearly, which would later be diagnosed by the AEA as a Communicative Handicap. It was her first label.

In the meantime, Rebecca's episodes of extreme physical aggression was turning our home into a battlefield. She had two methods of venting: the crying mode, where she was the only casualty, and the fury mode, where those in close proximity were the victims. Stephanie became an expert at spotting the warning signs and would alert me so I could run interference. When Rebecca went into fury mode, it was impossible to reason with her or calm her down, and I often became a human punching bag. To protect myself and subdue her, I had to grab her arms, pin them to her sides, and then quickly wrap my own arms around her tightly. After restraining her in a bear hug, I would carry her screaming and kicking upstairs to her bedroom. Once inside, I virtually had a split second to release her and run out, slamming the door shut behind me. She would beat on it and scream on one side while I sobbed and held tightly onto the knob from the other. It was emotionally devastating to listen to her screech and pound, but I knew of no other way to protect her, Stephanie, and myself from these violent outbursts. Being on the receiving end of Rebecca's tirades, I wanted to avoid the infliction of split lips, deep scratches, loss of hair, bent or broken glasses or being bitten. It was becoming increasingly more challenging to manage these episodes, and our lives were rapidly spinning out of control. I was terrified that one day *I* might lose control of my temper and hurt Rebecca.

You see, I intimately knew Rebecca's wrath because it also lurked deep within me. It had since I was as a teenager, and I knew how difficult it was to restrain that type of wildness. It has a short fuse, the velocity builds quickly, and the anger does not dissolve until it has been thoroughly spent. For many years, I had successfully kept it sealed and confined, but these situations were making that more and more difficult. Rebecca's bedroom door was the only thing protecting us from one another, and I could no longer ignore the fact that we desperately needed professional help.

As always, Rebecca finally quieted down, which meant that after destroying her room she had collapsed into an exhausted sleep and it was safe for me to release my tight grasp on her doorknob. One day, I turned from her door to find Stephanie silently watching from the safety of her own room across the hall. It wasn't the first time she had witnessed the demon that seemed to possess her little sister and my attempts to keep us safe, and it certainly wouldn't be the last. The rage that consumed Rebecca was uniting us in a way that no parent wishes to bond with their child. I pondered if the thoughts running through her mind were like those of my siblings who had witnessed my fits of anger.

On shaky legs, I went to Stephanie and wrapped her tightly in my arms. I offered her the same lame excuse of how we just needed to be patient with Rebecca until she could learn how to manage her temper. Hell, I certainly did not understand that madness when it suddenly appeared during my puberty years. Sure, I'd had moments of "Irish temperament" when I was younger, but it never had an extreme intensity or debilitating power until about age fifteen. Like Stephanie, some of my siblings had experienced similar episodes, when I was consumed by the monster and struck out at them. It was never my intention to hurt them, and thankfully they had an extraordinary capacity for forgiveness; however, the truth was that no amount of apologies could eliminate the pain my fury had inflicted. Now, as history repeated itself in my little girl, I realized that while I may have learned to suppress my ugly genetic blueprint, I'd never truly learned how to manage it. It was time to acknowledge that I could not teach what I did not know and start seeking a solution that would diffuse this escalating situation, protect both girls and make our lives peaceful again.

At the same time, I also had to do what I could to nurture the bond between Stephanie and Rebecca. Stephanie both loved and feared her sister, emotions I could certainly relate to; she also understood that Rebecca did not mean to hurt either of us. No matter how busy or overwhelmed I was, I made sure that Stephanie felt secure and confident in my love so she could honestly share her feelings. I listened, comforted, and tried to reassure her that things would be okay in time. It was vital for our family's unity that we always love one another, support one another, and be dedicated to one another, most especially during difficult times.

My vision of a supportive family did not include physical discipline. This was not just a philosophical belief, however, but one born of experience and fear that I would lose control. Given my own demon's ugly capacity for inflicting tremendous physical and emotional pain, oftentimes before I even realized it had come out, my version of "spanking" never went beyond a quick swat to the girls' behinds to get their attention. I held true to this even during Rebecca's worst moments, and other than the bear hug restraint I did not use physical measures to control her.

There will always be a debate regarding the pros and cons of spanking; some, like my parents and their parents before them, believe it is a valid form of discipline. Mom and Dad felt spanking was not only an acceptable form of punishment, but something of a parental obligation to deter unwanted behavior and teach right from wrong. It was their method, but it was never mine. In my opinion, hitting teaches hitting. It is as simple as that. One only needs to observe children at play as they "reprimand" their toys by hitting or making angry statements. Where do we suppose they learned to mimic that behavior?

Today's parents have what past generations did not: access to an abundance of statistics regarding parenting techniques that do not include physical intervention. My approach to parenting was that it was my responsibility to be my children's teacher. They came into the world innocent babies, and my every interaction with them was going to leave a lasting impression, regardless of my intent. That made me accountable for being the best parent I knew how to be with the skills I had. I acquired these skills largely by watching other parents, and when I saw something I admired I would then incorporate it into my own parenting style. The battle to control my temper was an ongoing effort, and one I was very committed to. I had learned personally, and painfully, that nothing productive ever comes from anger, and that physical abuse is just as damaging to the body as mental abuse is to the mind.

From the beginning, Greg and I decided that we would be consistent when dealing with the girls, and that we would always present to them a united front so they couldn't play one parent against the other. (Of course, Greg would reduce his accountability by always saying "Go ask Mom" when the girls wanted him to make a decision.) We strived to build a strong, loving, and respectful relationship with our girls and taught by example. Each of us was accountable for our actions, the words we spoke, and the pain we inflicted. There were no double standards, and honesty was the only way to build trust. We treated others in the way we wished to be treated and made sure the girls understood that all decisions came with good or bad consequences.

When Rebecca woke up from her mayhem, I once again explained to her why her behavior was unacceptable. She would apologize to her sister and then to me with gentle hugs and soft words of genuine regret, which made it easy for us to forgive her and begin the healing process yet again. After the apologies, she then began to clean up the destruction in her room created during her Tasmanian moment, while I prayed the police didn't show up at our door to investigate. The houses in our neighborhood sat relatively close to one another, and as we could hear our neighbors I knew they most likely heard the screams and banging from our home. Thankfully, we were spared that particular humiliation.

That evening, Greg came from work only to find himself standing in a minefield. Though it had ended sometime earlier, I was still distressed from Rebecca's latest eruption and unfortunately poor Greg got blasted. It was difficult for him to understand my exasperation as he had yet to witness the intensity of rampages – those she reserved for me and her sister. After hearing about it secondhand, all he could do was sternly talk to her about being "naughty" and tell her not to do it again. It irritated me immensely that she could control herself around him, and that she was intimidated by him and not by me.

Finally, one day, Rebecca lost control and had a mild temper tantrum in front of him. The boom of his voice as he bellowed for her to knock it off scared the heck out of both of us; this was followed by the sharp snap of his fingers. Rebecca stopped immediately, as if her father wielded some immense power from his pointing index finger. The simplicity with which he had handled her both infuriated me and made me feel like an inferior parent, though this was certainly not his intent. He was only doing what dads do - being the hammer! How could I be so proficient at parenting and disciplining Stephanie and fail so miserably where Rebecca was concerned?

After spending some time beating myself up over this, I shared my feelings with Mom, who, as usual, helped me gain perspective. She explained that even in this day and age the majority of childrearing often falls to the mother, and because we're around so much kids learn to block out our voice. That was the reason she had said, "Wait until your dad gets home!" to curtail unruly behavior when my siblings and I were young.

Hearing this gave me a much better understanding of my own family's dynamic. Greg worked hard to support us, which meant he had much less time to spend with the girls than I did but was a more effective disciplinarian when he was around. Though I certainly worked hard as well, I was also very fortunate to be able to stay home and develop a more intimate relationship with the girls; however, it was because of this relationship that Rebecca knew what my buttons were and the opportunity to push them. To help supplement our income, I did provide daycare for some of my nieces and nephews, and later would add waitressing a couple nights a week as well.

The battles with Rebecca continued to escalate until one day, while I was trying to subdue her, she struck me with such astonishing force that my glasses went flying, and I tasted blood from the split in my lip. I was so stunned I could not prepare for her second attack of curled fingers, aiming for my eyes. Survival instinct took over and without thinking, I pushed her away with the palm of my hand, knocking her back into her bedroom. I then quickly slammed the door shut, and held on for dear life to that doorknob, crying and praying that I had not hurt her, yet I still could not let go of the knob to check. When she was finally quiet, I raced downstairs and made a frantic phone call to the local Mental Health Office. My whole body was shaking as I divulged to the woman on the other end about the dangerous situation escalating in our home and my desperate need for immediate assistance.

Confident that she was going to provide support, I was shocked to hear her say that due to Rebecca's inability to carrying on an in-depth conversation, she was unable to help us at that time. Once Rebecca was able to communicate better, she added, I was welcome to call back. Was she kidding me? Here I was pleading for help, and she was turning me down! This dense fog seemed to squeeze the air out of my chest, paralyzing my ability to process any further thought. Sliding down the wall to the kitchen floor, I sobbed. We were doomed, I thought as the despair pulled me in like quicksand, and honestly, in that moment I had no desire to save myself.

Fear, disillusion, loneliness, and loss of faith came crashing down on me. I felt entirely abandoned and isolated from the rest of the world. I don't know how long I sat there until the deluge of tears passed and a pounding headache compelled me to get up off the floor to take some aspirin. What I do know is that as I sat, curled up as small as I could make myself and wishing for death, I heard a whisper reminding me of the promise I'd made to God in the delivery room. I had begged and promised to accept any complications if Rebecca's life was spared, and though it was made under horrific circumstances, it was not made lightly. Shame filled my mind, followed by determination. It was inconceivable not to honor my word, and therefore, self-pity was not an option. Drying my tears, I prayed harder, asking God to give me the determination and show me the direction for attaining help for Rebecca.

CHAPTER THREE

The Desperate Search for Knowledge

"There are two ways to slide easily through life: to believe everything or to doubt everything. Both ways save us from thinking."

Alfred Korzybski

As painful as it was, crying that river of tears had released an enormous weight of pent-up emotions that had held me captive since the day Rebecca was born. By this time, her sporadic physical outbursts had reached a point where taking her out in public was almost impossible. Her screams and physical assaults provoked distasteful looks of condemnation from people and even a few comments like "That child needs a good spanking" or "That is one spoiled little girl." These individuals knew absolutely nothing about my abilities as a mother and felt entitled to make judgmental comments. Their criticisms should not have had the power to hurt me, but they did because I had already done a thorough job of beating myself up.

One time, after Mass, my cousin Kevin commented, "I know you have another daughter, but I never see her with you!" His innocent observation was a direct assault to my already floundering self-esteem, and it was too painful to admit to him, or anyone, that I was incapable of handling my younger child. Instead, I used humor to camouflage my pain and replied that I feared to bring her to church because sometimes she acts possessed by the devil. We laughed, and I quickly escaped with Stephanie. A swift departure had become my defense, and the smile and jokes were merely part of my protective armor. It was the self-inflicted belief that everyone judged my parenting skills with Rebecca and found me deficient that caused me profound pain. Heck, I thought it myself, so it was easy to imagine that it was their opinion as well.

I had embraced the naïve notion that if I just loved the girls deeply enough, it would make me successful in the motherhood department. Although this was a commendable goal, it was unrealistic and incredibly devastating. It was that purging of tears that, for the first time, enabled me to consider the possibility that what was happening with Rebecca was not entirely my fault. I had been successful in teaching Stephanie to be well-behaved, and I had tried to employ those same methods with Rebecca, with completely different results. Given the trauma of her birth and the early health issues she had faced, it stood to reason that something deeper, something beyond my parenting, was going on with Rebecca. I realized, that somewhere along the line, I had silenced the inner voice I had relied on most of my life.

My misguided sense of embarrassment and powerlessness had become obstacles that hindered my ability to manage Rebecca. Conceding to the possibility that the problems were not a reflection of my inadequacies enabled me to recognize that I was not a bad mother; I simply lacked the skills to help her. There was no shame in asking for help, only in denying that I needed any. Giving up the blame game empowered me to focus my attention on finding a solution for the turbulence threatening to destroy our family. My search brought me back to the Arrowhead Education Agency (AEA), where I had taken Rebecca regarding her hearing. At that time, I was unaware of their diversified departments that offered invaluable assistance to children with physical, learning, and mental disabilities.

This time, when I called for assistance there were no hesitation or regrets; I was given an appointment no questions asked. These services provided by the AEA were at no expense to us pursuant to Public Law 94-142, enacted in 1975, and section 504 of the Rehabilitation Act of 1973, which is a civil rights law. Public Law 94-142 concerns learning disabilities involving speaking or understanding language, as well as listening, spelling, writing, or the ability to perform math skills. Section 504 of the Rehabilitation Act of 1973 protects the disabled in any agency that accepts federal funding from discrimination because of their handicap. You can contact the principal or superintendent of your school district for more information regarding the services provided in your area.

At our appointment, I found the staff to be polite, informative, professional, and compassionate about our fears and nervousness. The process involved an interview with me and Rebecca and another with me alone, followed by a series of evaluations on Rebecca to determine if she met the necessary criteria to qualify for assistance. Rebecca was relaxed and cooperative during her testing, but I found it very uncomfortable to be so closely scrutinized by these professionals. During my interview, I worried that they were going to proclaim me unfit, not only as a mom but also as a human being. My primary fear was that they would unearth my guarded secret: that I harbored continual and tremendous guilt regarding Rebecca's birth. Though my doctor had repeatedly reassured me that it was not my fault, I could not absolve myself from the liability that my body had created the rapid delivery that ultimately inflicted her trauma.

It was about a month later when we returned to the AEA for Rebecca's results. As I joined the staff in the conference room, I had a moment of foreboding and regret that I had not insisted that Greg attend. Each person took their turn explaining the test they had given Rebecca and their findings. I listened intently to the difficulties she had exhibited, then heard the diagnosis of "Communicative Handicap," which, as mentioned earlier, regarded her trouble processing information and its impact on her language skills. They also found that Rebecca had a significant delay in her motor skills. The combination and severity of these issues qualified her for home intervention. While sitting there processing their analyses, I felt a sense of relief and even optimism about finally having an explanation for Rebecca's behavior problems. However, these feelings quickly faded as the overall meaning of this new knowledge fully registered with my consciousness.

It was one thing to suspect a problem and quite another to have it so explicitly confirmed. These numerous obstacles would undoubtedly impede Rebecca from fitting in with society's realm of "normal"; instead, from this point forward, she would walk through life with the label of "disability." That reality check was both heartbreaking and terrifying for me because I had no idea of the nature or the extent of the difficulties she would have to endure. I tried to focus on comprehending the strategies and goals the team had put together to assist Rebecca, but it was a struggle to listen when my mind pulsated with humiliation that my body had created this brain injury that was now cheating her out of a normal life.

My Irish temperament desperately wanted to break or throw something in protest. No child should have to deal with issues like this! Greg had (and still does) teased that my best outcomes are usually when my temper has been fired up, and that day, I was mad as hell. After the meeting, I left Rebecca with Mom and went off by myself to rant and rave about the injustice. There would be countless venting episodes before I finally worked through my anger and grief for the loss of dreams that I had for Rebecca. Rationally, I knew what mattered most was acceptance of her diagnoses and staying focused on the challenges that would follow. Anything less would be a betrayal of my love for her. My emotions were a different story, though, and there would be many days when I leaned toward embracing a pity party.

Most of us can point to at least one person who has made significant impacts on their character and, for me, that person was Grandpa Ralph.

He was my paramount teacher, and I adored him. When I was about ten, he came upon me sitting on the back step complaining about something. He sat down beside me and patiently waited for my tirade to end, then he looked at me with those wise eyes of his and told me I had two choices in dealing with the hard knocks of life. I could pick myself up, dust off my britches, and continue with life, or I could dig a hole in the backyard and sit in it and feel sorry for myself. He explained that while I sat in that hole, life was going to pass on by, and he was not staying around to watch me dig a hole. In his infinite wisdom, Grandpa Ralph taught me that nothing productive ever came from wallowing in self-pity, and though I may never fully understand or appreciate the challenges I face, I try to follow his advice and dust off my britches. My motto became, "Fortunate are those of us who are only pricked by the thorns of life." In other words, there is always someone dealing with worse things than I am encountering or will encounter, so I strive to count my blessings instead of my woes.

The AEA assigned Margo as Rebecca's home intervention teacher, and she would come once a week to work with Rebecca on communication and comprehension skills, as well as her inappropriate behavior. On her first visit, Margo explained the goals they had set for Rebecca, then addressed the disciplinary problems I was experiencing. She described the "timeout" technique and wanted me to use it full time, rather than just for Rebecca's extreme temper tantrums. The premise was that consistently using this behavioral management strategy would discourage unwanted behavior. I was extremely skeptical of the effectiveness of sitting Rebecca in a chair for the timeout, and I said as much to Margo. Hell, the only way I had been able to keep her in her room during a rage was by holding the door shut.

For those who may not know about this method of discipline, it works like this: you sit the child in a chair and, depending on the child's age and severity of the infraction, set the limit for timeout, usually from two to five minutes. If the child is extremely aggressive, then the timeout is restricted to the bedroom and set at five to ten minutes. For this disciplinary action to be successful, you first need to explain to the child that the "timeout" is the result of his or her inappropriate behavior; then you instruct them to sit quietly in the chair for the predetermined time. The timeout does not begin until they are quiet and calm.

The second part of this technique, which is nonnegotiable, is that you do not enter into an argument or a discussion with your child after placing him/her in the timeout. By eliminating all conversation, you take control of the situation away from the child and place it into your hands where it belongs. If your child refuses to sit in the chair for the timeout, you continually put them in the chair until they remain seated. Use the same procedure for a timeout in the bedroom. By consistently using this technique, you prevail over your child's stubbornness and eliminate their power to manipulate you and the situation. The objective of this strategy is to hold the child accountable for their actions and, ultimately, teaches them consequences.

Margo and I discussed Rebecca's strengths, weakness, difficulties, manipulative behavior and outbursts. Although I had forewarned Margo about Rebecca's considerable skill at manipulation, I knew she would be unable to comprehend the depth of this character trait until she knew Rebecca better. Yes, it is normal for children to use manipulation to get their way, but our daughter had turned it into an artform. That charming smile of hers and the allure of innocence could con the devil out of his pitchfork! The moment finally arrived to introduce Rebecca, and I called her down from upstairs. She descended the stairs with her sweetest smile in place and just the right pretense of bashfulness, and I knew Margo was about to become the fly in the spider's web.

Rebecca sat down on the couch between us, avoiding eye contact with me as she watched Margo pull out some toys, puzzles, and shapes of all sizes from her bag of goodies. I quietly observed as Margo placed the items on the table in front of Rebecca, then gave her directions. Rebecca listened attentively, then performed each task just as Margo requested, and it was difficult to ascertain whether the tests and new toys genuinely enthralled her or she was playing her usual mind games.

My intuition leaned toward the latter. The hour ended and Margo asked Rebecca to help put the toys back into the bag, and I thought, oh boy, here it comes. She had been perfectly content playing with all the new toys, and now, Margo was asking her to relinquish them.

Here was just the type of scenario that provoked her temper, so I prepared for the outburst and was flabbergasted when she willingly complied by helping to put the toys back in the bag. Who was this little girl? When Margo got ready to leave, she praised Rebecca for her hard work and cooperation and made an appointment to return the following week. We walked Margo to the door, and while watching as she walked to her car, I glanced down at Rebecca and thanked her for good behavior. She looked up at me with that familiar smirk and laughed wickedly as she ran upstairs to play. Well, that was all the verification that I needed that Margo - and to some extent myself - had been deceived by her facade of compliance.

I thought Rebecca would surely lose it during Margo's second visit, but once again she was the picture of charm and composure. Then, on the third visit, the inevitable happened. Margo asked Rebecca to put the last toy in the bag, and my little darling refused to surrender her new treasure. When Margo extended her hand and made a second request, Rebecca just tightened her grip, a sure sign that a battle was about to ensue. I interceded at this point and firmly told Rebecca to give Margo the toy, and as anticipated, she refused so I pried it from her fingers of steel and handed it to Margo. The squall began, and the storm of rage quickly followed.

Rebecca let loose her scream of outrage and began hitting and kicking me, so I proceeded to follow through with the timeout technique that I had regularly been using. As soon as I placed her in the chair, my little yo-yo child bounced right back out, swinging and kicking at me. Margo watched in horror at Rebecca's unleashed anger and refusal to remain in the chair. Fearful of losing my own temper, I decided to remove her from the situation. When she bounced out again, I picked her up and carried her screaming and kicking the entire way upstairs. I put her down in her bedroom, shut the door, but thankfully no longer needed to hold the door closed. That much progress had been made by using the timeout method. It took a few moments to compose myself and gather my courage before going downstairs to face Margo.

I expected to be chastised for not following through, but Margo was utterly shocked and deeply disturbed by how quickly Rebecca had become violent. Her reaction to Rebecca's rage mirrored others who had witnessed our small hurricane in action. No amount of warning or description could ever prepare people for the existence of Rebecca's dark side, not after seeing only her friendly disposition. The full realization of her aggressive nature, or the velocity of her anger, came only from witnessing it for the first time. Astounded and speechless was always the reactions and, if it were not such a dire situation, I would have found their expressions humorous.

One memory that stands out was the day I invited Dena, who had recently become my friend, to go shopping with Rebecca and myself. Although Dena had heard about Rebecca's nasty temper, she had never observed more than a mild attitude from my daughter. That all changed the day at the mall. What had been a pleasurable outing quickly deteriorated when we started approaching the outside doors and Rebecca realized we were leaving. She began dragging her heels and attempted to pull her hand free from mine, so I tighten my grip, which prompted the hitting. Knowing a fight was unavoidable, I tried to pick her up, but she thwarted my maneuver, threw herself on the floor, and lay there screaming and kicking. Dodging her thrashing arms and legs, I managed to get a firm grip around her middle and lifted her off the floor with my usual bear hug. Of course, this wrestling match only increased the volume of her screams as she fought harder against the confinement. Using my back, I pushed the door open to get outside and looked at the people standing there, staring at us as if we were a freak show at the circus. Poor Dena was standing there with her mouth hanging open in total astonishment.

Rebecca continued to create a scene as I carried her to the car. Finally, exhausted, she stopped screaming and struggling as her protest turned to silent tears. When we reached the car, she climbed in and sat down in her car seat while I secured the safety latch. She looked up at me with those beautiful blue eyes with tears rolling down her face and, my anger and embarrassment instantly dissolved. It was tormenting to watch these tirades consume her, and the misery in her eyes afterward was more devastating than any physical pain she inflicted. Rebecca was utterly lost during these episodes, and once the cloud of distress cleared, she seemed confused, disoriented, and thoroughly drained. People's stares and unkind comments were temporary discomforts compared to the emotional turmoil that Rebecca endured. I would have given anything if my little girl could be calm and happy.

When Dena finally caught up with us, I apologized for the embarrassment she must have felt, but her main concern was for my welfare from the physical abuse Rebecca inflicted. She did admit to being somewhat shocked that a thing as inconsequential as leaving the mall could cause such a violent reaction. Rather than impart judgment or criticism, Dena attempted to lighten the mood with her unique gift of humor, and her genuine compassion and lack of judgment sealed our bond of friendship. She became my much-needed lifeline to sanity, and from that day forward continues to bless my life as one of my greatest supporters.

After Margo witnessed Rebecca's outburst, she felt a professional intervention would be beneficial and planned to bring Carl, a child psychologist, on her next visit. She was hopeful that he would be able to provide valuable and appropriate techniques for managing Rebecca's behavioral disorder. Carl attended the next session and performed tests similar to those Margo had administered. Once again, Rebecca was polite and cooperative during the evaluation. When she finished, Carl congratulated her on a job well done and told her she could go play. Carl could not find any problems since Rebecca had been cooperative, but Margo expressed concern over her struggles with several of the tests. I agreed with her feedback, and noted that Rebecca had easily completely nearly identical tests when Margo had given them. We questioned whether

Rebecca had truly forgotten how to do them or if she was performing for Carl's benefit.

Due to our concerns, Carl agreed that further observation would be helpful and planned to attend the following week to see if Rebecca exhibited aggressive or manipulative actions. As I feared, Rebecca maintained extraordinary self-control again in Carl's presence, and it made me wonder if she somehow understood what his title meant. She only portrayed the sweet and adorable side of her personality and seemed to be intentionally avoiding any opportunity for him to discover signs of her temperament or manipulation skills. It made me truly grateful that Margo had witnessed her at her explosive worst and could validate my declaration that Rebecca seemed to possess this Jekyll and Hyde personality.

In the meantime, I continued to implement the timeout procedure each day, with Rebecca remaining resilient in her fight against this disciplinary action. As soon as I placed her in the chair she would spring back out, then, just when I was ready to admit defeat, Rebecca shocked the heck out of me and stayed in the chair! She still protested at the top of her lungs, but it was definitely cause for celebration. The next challenge was getting her to remain silent when placed in the timeout. Although I had doubted this strategy would work with Rebecca, I am so happy that I persevered and did not let discouragement win. It took consistency and extreme patience but was well worth the effort and time. Within a few months, I only had to instruct Rebecca to go to timeout and she would sit quietly in the chair. Gone was her need to manipulate me into a conversation or dismantle her room, and I was ecstatic over this incredible progress.

I had a newfound respect for the staff members of the AEA, whose expertise, dedication, and compassion spared our family from further deterioration. As Rebecca approached her fourth birthday, Greg and I contemplated sending her to preschool. I discussed this option with Margo who supported our decision and so Rebecca was enrolled at a neighboring school three days a week from nine to eleven-thirty a.m.

The night before her first day, Greg and I joked that in all likelihood, our daughter would be the first kid ever to be kicked out of preschool. Rebecca was very excited on her first day, and when she got to the classroom, there were no tears, fears or waves goodbye as she quickly ran to check out the new surroundings. When I returned to pick her up, she was enthusiastic about her experience and wanted to go out to lunch and celebrate.

We had been home less than fifteen minutes when the phone rang, and I was engaged in a serious conversation with Rebecca's teacher. She was very apologetic, but she felt that our daughter was challenging and perhaps it would be better if we found a different school. Well, the joke was on us! Rebecca was being kicked out of preschool on the first day.

Heartbroken, I called Margo to let her know about the teacher's evaluation, and she said she would consult with Carl and call me back. The two of them contacted the teacher on Rebecca's behalf and persuaded her to allow Rebecca to come back to class for just the first hour. Margo and Carl would offer support in helping Rebecca adjust to the expectations of a classroom environment. The hope was that in time, she would return to class for the regularly scheduled time. Several weeks into this joint effort, I arrived early to peek undetected through the window, and what I observed was greatly disheartening. All the students were sitting on the floor in a circle as the teacher chased after Rebecca, politely requesting her to join the other children. Ignoring the teacher, she headed over to a shelf and pulled down a toy, which the teacher took away and put back on the shelf. Rebecca, being an obstinate little bugger, stepped around the teacher and took a different toy down as the other children sat quietly watching.

Then two boys jumped up and left the circle to join Rebecca and play with the toys. The teacher was noticeably flustered at not being able to redirect Rebecca's attention but was successful at getting the boys to return to the circle. Sadly, our little terror had tasted power and would fight to the bitter end for control of that classroom. There was only one option: I opened the door and walked in. Everyone turned to look at me, including the teacher, whose relief was palpable. I gave Rebecca my "squint-eyed look of displeasure," which she knew well, then firmly instructed her to put the toy away, apologize to her teacher, and stand by the door. Once she had apologized, I then did the same and walked out the door with Rebecca in tow.

With Rebecca's refined skills at manipulation and her intense need to be in control, she enjoyed treating people as if they were opponents in her little game. It was as though she had this superpower to look directly into a person's soul, size them up, and then play them like an accomplished musician. Softhearted people with easygoing personalities became putty in her hands as she either thoroughly charmed them or wickedly harassed them. Unfortunately, her teacher was a gentle soul and therefore, did not stand a chance against our daughter's masterful skills. If a person had a strong personality, Rebecca was instinctively cautious and gave them grudging respect, except where I was concerned. She was not only proficient at trying my limited patience; she also attained great satisfaction from challenging me. The paramount obstacles in our relationship were our strong personalities, and both of us were fighting for control.

After what I had witnessed in class, it was evident that this preschool was not going to work. I had the utmost respect, admiration, and appreciation for this teacher agreeing to work with the AEA, but her passive personality was no match for Rebecca. Her negative behavior made class time unproductive, and as disheartening as it was, we decided that it was in everyone's best interest to remove Rebecca from preschool. I called the teacher, who sounded relieved to hear the news, and then Margo, who was genuinely disappointed about our decision. A few days later, Margo called to set up an appointment for her and Carl to visit and discuss Rebecca's inability to function in a regular classroom environment.

During that visit Carl broached the possibility of using medication to treat her "hyperactivity"; it was the first time I had heard that word used to describe my daughter's behavior. This revelation was unsettling to say the least, as was the suggestion that we medicate her. I learned that a drug called Ritalin was quite often effective in calming these children and improving their ability to learn in the classroom. I asked if the Ritalin would cure the hyperactivity, and he informed me that there was no known cure.

As I listened to Carl, my first reaction was one of anger. It was one thing to admit that Rebecca was extremely active, overly excitable, and prone to throwing temper tantrums, but quite another to label her hyperactive. Again, this was 1988, the "dark ages" when it came to the accessibility of information; therefore, my perception of hyperactive kids came from the opinions of others. They were considered abnormal, a menace to society, oddballs, bullies, sugar junkies, and little monsters only a mother could love.

Of course, Carl had no way of knowing how I felt or, how difficult it had been for me to accept that my daughter had a Communitive Handicap. Now, as he sat at our kitchen table, calmly adding yet another diagnosis, it was like he was adding salt to a freshly mended wound. His suggestion of using a drug to modify Rebecca's behavior to meet the expectations of preschool was just too much. Things were not that simple for me, and I was not going to comply based solely on his opinion, professional as it may be.

Rebecca was four years old and to use a medication for an incurable and non-life-threatening disorder made very little sense. When Carl was unable to answer some of my questions regarding Ritalin, I decided to educate myself on the drug, and on hyperactivity in general. My search began at our local library, with the daunting task of looking through index catalogs. For those of you who don't remember, they were tall wood cabinets with many drawers, each with a letter of the alphabet on the outside. Inside were index cards, each with the title of a book and a summary of its information. Several nights a week, I would bathe the girls so they would be ready to tuck in for the night and then head off to the library.

The books and materials available for my research were somewhat limited and written mostly by physicians or researchers. A few magazine articles were available, but most of the information I found seemed to have conflicting opinions as to the cause and treatment for ADHD. What I failed to discover, and desperately needed, was something written by a parent offering their perspective on how they survived the turmoil of raising a hyperactive child. I was looking for a handbook of techniques to guide me, offer me hope, and give me a sense of unity, rather than the isolation I had been feeling. Some nights, my brain got so tired from reading that it would painfully protest like a drum solo.

The more material I devoured, the more overwhelmed and conflicted I became. My intention to seek data had created two additional challenges. Not only did I have to make sense of all this new knowledge, I had to figure out how best to utilize it to benefit Rebecca. Just about every book or paper on ADHD mentioned the use of Ritalin as treatment, and many authors supported it or similar drugs for treatment. The issue for me, however, was the serious side effects, potential health risks, and the possibility for additional medicines becoming necessary for continued effectiveness. Reading this information made me particularly apprehensive and reinforced my belief that drug therapy to manage the symptoms of ADHD was not in Rebecca's best interest. There was no mention in any resource I found of implementing an all-natural diet as an alternative to medication. In all probability, if I had not so thoroughly researched Ritalin, I might have assumed it was a suitable option. During the course of my research, however, I had discovered several red flags and I could not disregard them, no matter how badly I wanted a solution.

After careful consideration, I decided to forgo medication and continue instead with behavior modification, the plan being to revisit preschool the following year. Needing validation that I had made the correct decision, I went to see mom, hoping that the insight and wisdom she had gained from raising nine kids would apply to this situation. As usual, Mom did not disappoint. After telling me she also did not support using medication to treat Rebecca, she presented me with a gift: a book called *Why Your Child is Hyperactive by Dr. Ben Feingold*. Though by this time considerable progress had been made using behavior modification,

Mom obviously felt a need for this book and had been waiting for an opportunity to give it to me. As she placed it in my hand, she expressed confidence in my ability to find the best solutions for my daughter. Mom had always been my devoted cheerleader, and no, I was not smart enough to read the book.

When I got home, I called Margo to let her know that I was not comfortable medicating Rebecca, and though she may not have agreed with my choice, she respected my wishes and offered continued support. A few days later, Margo called and asked me to join her on a visit to the Developmental Learning Center (DLC). The DLC was an environment for children with various disabilities and possibly had a place for Rebecca. Margo picked us up the next morning and we settled in at the back of Sheryl's classroom to observe. It was surprising to see the range of disabilities among the children, and when I glanced at Rebecca to gauge her reaction, I found her intently watching.

There were children who, like Rebecca, showed no outward signs of a disability, and others with varying degrees of mental and physiological disabilities. Sheryl was truly awe-inspiring, with her natural and easy way of addressing their academic and physical needs. She had a genuine ability to connect with her students, and they responded well to her directions and authority and appeared to be comfortable within their surroundings. The rest of the staff was also impressive as they balanced each child's challenges and unique gifts. Still, I was not entirely convinced that the DLC was the right choice for Rebecca. The ride back home was a quiet one. Margo seemed to understand and respect that my lack of conversation was most likely due to me trying to process what I had observed.

Later that night, in the quiet darkness after saying my prayers, it came to me that I still had a hidden layer of denial regarding Rebecca's disabilities. Despite everything I had experienced, I kept clinging to the idea that if I just worked hard enough she would overcome the obstacles fate had dealt her. That illusion had largely been shattered by my visit to the DLC and my acceptance that the severity of Rebecca's disabilities warranted her placement there. Now, with deep sorrow, I finally surrendered to the knowledge that my little girl was destined to encounter endless struggles and pain throughout her life. Not only would she have to endure the hard work necessary to withstand her disabilities, she would also have to persevere against the prejudice and cruelty of society. I am not sure if people are just uncomfortable, incapable of comprehending, lacking in empathy, or simply do not care, but many are incredibly unkind to those with disabilities, especially children. Individuals who do not fit into the preconceived realm of "normalcy" are far too often looked upon as a secondary class of humanity. These deeply ingrained shortcomings in our society will always be a concern for Greg and me with regard to how people look at and treat Rebecca.

Because Greg was unable to attend our visit to the DLC, he relied entirely upon my instincts about whether to send Rebecca there. It was an enormous responsibility to carry alone, and I feared how placing Rebecca in this environment would ultimately affect her self-image. She saw life through the eyes of an innocent four-year-old who was completely unaware that she even had disabilities. When she looked in the mirror, the reflection she identified with was that of a little girl whose mannerisms and speech made perfect sense. How would I live with myself if placing her in the DLC shattered that innocence? I also worried how she would interpret this new environment, adapt to school on a full-time basis, and adjust to the long bus ride. In the end, I had to set aside my uncertainties and do whatever I could to ensure that Rebecca had every opportunity to reach her full potential in life.

With a leap of faith and trust in the Lord, we decided that Rebecca, with her fighting spirit and tenacity, could persevere anything if she just wanted it bad enough. I also trusted that Sheryl was the teacher capable of addressing Rebecca's academic needs and handling her strong personality. Sheryl had demonstrated an extraordinary patience, a positive nature, and an unshakable belief that children with special needs were capable of learning if their individual needs were addressed.

On her first day of class at the DLC, Rebecca was excited as we waited for the bus on the front sidewalk. When it arrived, she eagerly climbed the stairs, turned, and smiled at me, and then found a seat next to a window. With a huge smile, she waved as the bus pulled away and I waved back with both a smile and tears running down my face. It depressed me that Rebecca was leaving on a big yellow bus and would spend six and a half hours a day, five days a week at school. However, my sadness was more about her not experiencing the typical traditions of childhood like the ones her sister did.

Rebecca's transition into the DLC began smoothly, and she appeared to be adjusting well to the rules and expectations. Sheryl, like Margo, was supportive of open communication and encouraged my input regarding my knowledge of Rebecca's temperament and behaviors. Things seemed to be on track and reinforced our confidence that we had found the perfect school. It was a few months later that Rebecca got off the bus crying, raced up to me angry, and demanded to know why I had not told her that she was retarded! My greatest fear had just been realized, and Rebecca was enduring pain and cruelty from someone who used an ugly word as an insult. Some boy on the bus told her that she was mentally retarded, and now all I could do was tightly wrap my arms around her and try to give comfort as she cried.

I knew this was just the first of many painful situations we would encounter in her life, and this coupled with the knowledge that there was little I could do to protect her, was agonizing. As soon as she settled down, I asked why she believed what a total stranger said to her. Never had I discussed the trauma of her birth with her, but the day had arrived to tell Rebecca about God helping our doctor save her life. She listened intently, and then I explained to her that only God knows what each of us can achieve in our life. I admitted that her brain, like mine, just worked differently than some people and that only meant that we both had to work harder to learn things. She seemed to process this information and then kissed my cheek and went off to play. It would be the first of many times that we bonded over tears from hateful words or actions done to her just because she had been born different.

One peaceful afternoon, I received a call from the school informing me that Rebecca was exhibiting disruptive behaviors in class. The reprieve was over, and Carl had been called for a consultation. After observing Rebecca, he suggested that Sheryl use a number system as an effective strategy to correct her disregard for compliance. She would start the day with ten numbers, and each infraction would result in her losing a number. If Rebecca reached number five, Sheryl was to send her to the office, where the secretary would put Rebecca on the phone to tell me about her inappropriate behavior. I made it clear to Rebecca that this would be her only warning. If after returning to the classroom she lost any more numbers, a privilege would be taken away at home, a consequence she disliked immensely.

This form of behavioral management worked relatively well in making things quiet on the school front once again. However, like all the other strategies we had come up with, it eventually began to fail. The verbal reminders and loss of privileges became less of a deterrent to keep Rebecca on track, and the next call was from Sheryl asking if I had any suggestions.

I did not, but I assured her that I was off to the library to find us a new behavioral technique and would call her back after the weekend. What I came across was another method incorporating the use of numbers, but with a significant difference. This strategy allowed the child to earn back numbers with good behavior, which provided them an opportunity of redemption after using poor judgment. When I called Sheryl to share this encouraging new discovery, she told me that another teacher had suggested this very option to her. We decided she would implement it immediately.

Rebecca responded well to the revised strategy, and it bought us about another month before it too began to fail. The next phone call was not from Sheryl, but the school office and a request that I immediately pick up Rebecca. When I arrived, I saw Rebecca sitting in a chair and swinging her legs back and forth as if she did not have a care in the world. She saw me coming, smiled sweetly, and waved, which confirmed my suspicion that she had no idea the severity of the situation. As Sheryl was in class, a woman I had never met before told me she was sorry but until I corrected Rebecca's behavior she could not return to class. Rebecca's constant disruptive behavior prevented the other students from getting their work done and would no longer be tolerated. For the second time, Rebecca was being expelled from school!

While I was still trying to process the disbelief, she asked if my husband and I had ever considered placement in a facility better equipped to handle children with severe disruptive behaviors such as Rebecca. That comment was like a second slug to my gut, and I literally stood there staring at her with my mouth hanging open. When I found my voice, I asked the unthinkable: was she referring to an *institution*? She said it was more like a group home for children with extreme issues. She quickly followed up with the comment that we would be able to visit and take her home on weekends. What the hell? Was she serious? To say I was appalled that she even proposed such a thing was an understatement. As if removing Rebecca from our home and placing her in that type of environment would ever be an option! How anyone could believe taking our four-year-old child from her home and placing her with strangers, regardless of their credentials, was beneficial was beyond my comprehension.

Resisting the urge to punch the woman in the face, I instead grabbed Rebecca's hand and we stormed off down the long dim hallway toward the exit, then into the bright sunshine outside. I had no idea what we were going to do now that the DLC was threatening to revoke their support. Somehow, I needed to find an immediate fix to her behavioral problems. Even as I thought this, something started tugging at my conscience. Either I was going to stand by my convictions that drug therapy was not in her best interest, or I was going to buckle under pressure and put her on Ritalin so she could stay in school. Honestly, in that moment I wanted to take the easy way out, give her the damn medication, and make all our lives easier.

I cried the whole way across town to my mom's, with Rebecca asking me repeatedly what the matter was. My world was once again spinning out of control, and I just needed to see Mom and hear her agree that medication was indeed the only solution. However, when I told her about the situation at school and that I was thinking of using the drug, she immediately asked me if I'd even read the book she had given me. When I replied, "Not yet," she gave me a look of disgust and told me to go home and read the damn book! As I drove down the street, I saw three of my brothers standing outside the local convenience store and pulled in hoping that once I shared my horrible experience, they would give me the sympathy Mom had not. One brother had no advice, the second believed I would do the right thing, and the third thought I should follow the opinion of the experts; if they thought placement was best for Rebecca. None of those answers told me what I wanted to hear, so I got back in the car even more frustrated and cursed the sun for daring to shine when thunder and lightning were more in tune with my mood!

When we got home, Rebecca raced off to play while I began reading Dr. Feingold's book. The farther I got into the book, the more I wanted to kick my butt for not reading it right away. I had avoided doing so because I had assumed it would be dry and clinical, like everything else I'd read by doctors. Was I ever off base on that one! According to Dr. Feingold, I could change Rebecca's behavior simply by changing her diet. Armed with what I believed was a good strategy, I called to explain the Feingold Diet to Sheryl and ask for her support while I tried it. She was willing, she said, but first she had to get permission from her bosses for Rebecca to return to class. I hung up the phone both heartened by Sheryl's open-mindedness and terrified that the administrators would hold firm to Rebecca's expulsion. I honestly doubted I would survive mentally if they did.

CHAPTER FOUR

The Man behind the Diet

"There's no need to believe what an artist says. Believe what he does; that's what counts."

David Hockney

D r. Ben F. Feingold wrote *Why Your Child is Hyperactive* to help those suffering from allergies and an intolerance to certain foods and chemicals. Born, raised and educated in Pennsylvania, Dr. Feingold had started his medical career in the late 1920s, working in various hospitals in Germany, Austria and, finally, Los Angeles. He eventually specialized in allergy treatment of children, then later expanded his practice to include adults. Seeking a way to make a greater impact, Dr. Feingold left private practice in 1951 and joined Kaiser Foundation Hospital and Permanente Medical Group, and established allergy clinics in Northern California. One of his earliest case studies involved an investigation into fleas, as numerous patients in the Bay Area were suffering from fleabites.

The objective of the project was to discover a remedy and a defense against this problem, but first he needed to process a chemical substance called an allergen. Since no allergen from fleas existed, he contacted the California Academy of Science and inquired where he could locate about one million fleas. They directed him to contact the Communicable Disease Center of U. S. Public Health who recommended that he apply for a grant from the National Institute of Health. Getting the grant was essential for creating the Laboratory of Medical Entomology, Kaiser Foundation Research Institute, of which he became the director.

Dr. Feingold and the staff used a variety of fleas to generate about a million fleas per week. It makes me want to scratch just thinking about that many little buggers. Through this flea experimentation they discovered that a reaction from a fleabite was due to the hapten, a chemical in the flea's saliva that was low in molecular weight. A small amount of hapten would not produce an allergic or immune reaction, however, when it was combined with a more substantial molecular weight such as proteins in the human body, it did create an allergic reaction. From this data, they determined that the hapten from the fleabite mixed with the skin's collagen, which is a protein, would make an individual prone to react.

After discovering a connection between hapten and proteins of the human body, the next step was to study the body's immune reaction. The tests confirmed that chemicals used as additives in foods and drugs were "low- molecular compounds" which had the same ability as the hapten found in the saliva of fleas. Dr. Feingold theorized that these findings could relate to his patients who had shown "adverse reactions" to aspirin. Applying that theory, he suggested his patients avoid aspirin and the artificial color yellow #5, Tartrazine, being used in some medications. Further insight came from a report by Dr. W.B. Shelley in the Journal of American Medical Association, which stated that some natural foods with salicylate had similar properties to aspirin and therefore could cause a reaction for those who were sensitive.

During this time, Dr. Alice Friedman, a resident working with Dr. Feingold, mentioned a German study with a list of foods with salicylates. Utilizing all the information, Dr. Feingold created his "salicylate-free" diet, which entailed avoiding oranges, grapes, peaches, raspberries, apricots, cucumbers, tomatoes, prunes, aspirin, and the artificial color

Tartrazine. Before long, he would learn about seven chemicals in foods that had the same components of salicylates and revised his diet again. Then a study appeared in a medical journal stating that although aspirin and FD& C "Yellow 5" had no similar properties, both had induced a reaction in asthma patients. This latest development led Dr. Feingold to consider that this may be the reason why some of his patients were not achieving successful results while adhering to his newly modified diet.

At this point, Dr. Sergio Ferreira and Dr. John Vane, two pharmacologists from London, joined his research. They gave an update on the drug Indomethacin, which was being used for arthritis. It was linked to the same reactions on the physiological production of prostaglandins, a group of natural mediators in the body. (Yep, I too found this information a little difficult to follow or grasp, but it is essential so please bear with me.) Here was another statistic to corroborate Dr. Feingold's belief that compounds with no resemblance to aspirin were, in fact, capable of a "cross-react" and could induce a reaction for someone with sensitivities. Realizing that there were several thousand synthetic chemicals present in drugs and foods, Dr. Feingold again modified his "salicylate-free" diet. This revision became the "elimination diet" and required his patients to avoid aspirin and foods with salicylates, as well as all drugs and foods artificially dyed or flavored. Patients adhering to this newest revision showed impressive results, while still others failed to improve.

In 1965, a woman about forty years old came to the Kaiser-Permanente Medical Center with hives and swelling around her eyes and face. Dr. Feingold had allergy tests performed and when the results came back negative, he suspected that artificial dyes and flavors were responsible for her condition. He prescribed the Kaiser-Permanente Diet (K-P Diet), and within three days the patient notified him that she had experienced a favorable response to the diet and that her skin was returning to normal.

Several weeks later, Dr. Feingold got a call from the Chief of Psychiatry at Kaiser Permanente asking what treatment he had prescribed for this female patient. The woman, unbeknownst to Dr. Feingold, had been seeing the psychiatrist for the past two years for her aggressive and hostile behaviors toward her husband, family, and at her place of employment.

According to the psychiatrist, in just over two weeks, the woman's unfavorable behaviors had dissipated, which surprised Dr. Feingold because the patient had not confided to him about her psychotherapy. Curious after the conversation with the psychiatrist, he called the patient for a follow-up consultation. Her skin was clear, and she appeared healthy; she also shared that things had significantly improved at home and at work. She did mention that if she deviated at all from the diet her previous behaviors would return. As intriguing as this case was, Dr. Feingold had to consider the possibility that the change in her demeanor could merely be a coincidence. He was not aware of any instances where artificial dyes or flavors had affected a patient's conduct and thought her response to the diet might be psychological. However, he asked his staff to keep an eye out for similar cases.

Within the next couple of years, an assortment of adults and children saw Dr. Feingold with symptoms ranging from asthma, hives, itching, skin rashes, and "personality disturbances" that were possibly associated with artificial colors and dyes. Some of the children had been diagnosed hyperactive. He placed these patients on the K-P Diet, thinking it would help with whatever allergies they had. When he heard about improvements in behavior and academics while on the diet, it did not raise a flag because he was an allergist, not a behavioral specialist. Like many specialists, Dr. Feingold was not always up to date on other current health developments, therefore he was unaware of the rise of hyperactivity.

In March of 1968, Dr. Feingold prepared a document titled "Recognition of Food Additives as a Cause of Symptoms of Allergy." This report was the result of hundreds of patients diagnosed as being hypersensitive to synthetic dyes and flavors, and he wanted to alert others about the dangers of artificial additives. He presented his findings in Denver at the Twenty-fourth Annual Congress of the American College of Allergists, where he stressed the importance of placing the precise name of a chemical dye on the label of food products and prescriptions.

Dr. Feingold felt strongly that correctly labeling foods and pharmaceuticals would be beneficial for physicians and the public as it would prevent dangerous adverse reactions to those who were susceptible. He also shared that England had already implemented this mandate for all product labels.

In the United States, however, the requirement for labels at this time was "US Certified Color," a vague term that made it impossible for physicians or patients to avoid certain chemicals in prescriptions. Dr. Feingold believed this type of inappropriate labeling had the potential to jeopardize a patient's wellbeing. Although the allergists seemed highly receptive to his recommendation, there was little interest from other arenas. In the meantime, the reported cases of patients with adverse reactions to synthetic dyes and flavors continued to rise each month.

As of January 2013, the Nutrition Labeling & Education Act requires that all ingredients be listed on the labels. The standard practice of the FDA is for companies to provide proof that their product is safe with their petition. With the FDA approval, they do their best once the item is distributed to protect the consumers with controlled studies and monitoring.

In the 1960s, however, this development was still several decades in the future, and Dr. Feingold and his contemporaries continued to research the negative effects certain dyes and chemicals were having on those with sensitivities. Dr. Farr and Dr. Samter presented a compelling study which concluded that unfavorable reactions to aspirin was *non-allergic*. This finding was crucial for aspirin-sensitive patients who showed a reaction to artificial dyes and flavors. These individuals, regardless of age or hyperactivity, did not have a defense against artificial additives. What Dr. Feingold found most remarkable about this study was that fifteen years after he began his research with fleas, low-molecule compounds were still relevant.

By the end of the sixties, Dr. Feingold was suffering from an illness that required a couple of surgeries and a lengthy recovery period. Forced to reduce his workload, Feingold used the time to write about his experiences as a doctor and researcher; this would become the textbook *Introduction to Clinical Allergy*. It took him several years to complete and by that time he was thinking about retiring so he could tend to his flowers and perhaps travel. That was until the subject of Hyperactivity and Learning Disabilities (H-LD) caught his attention. The previous term for this disorder was Minimal Brain Dysfunction (MBD) or, as some teachers called it, Specific Learning Disability (SLD). Over the past eleven years, there had been negligible attention given to the subject, but by 1971 there were about thirty-five professional articles, books, and medical reports publicized.

By 1972, interest had begun to spread, appearing in newspapers, on the radio, and on TV; Life Magazine even dedicated seven pages about the estimated millions of H-LD children. Dr. Feingold was both distressed and perplexed upon hearing this news because he had been unaware that so many children were suffering with the disorder and/or forced to manage it with medication. Although he had treated a variety of disorders, he had little recollection of so many children with the H-LD profile. There had been children and teens with epilepsy, psychological issues and mental challenges, but only a minimal number of children with hyperkinetic (hyperactivity) disorder. It was concerning to hear about the despair of parents and teachers due to the sweeping rise of children battling this disorder.

The situation disturbed him enough that he put off his retirement and began examining what was essentially an epidemic. He found that the earliest mention of this type of disorder in print was 1896, when James Kerr, a school physician, wrote about a reading disorder in "intelligent children." The label brain-damaged began to be used more in 1935 and later changed to Minimal Brain Dysfunction. This current situation of H-LD children reminded Dr. Feingold of his experience in 1928 while a graduate student in Vienna. Since the United States did not customarily provide residencies for pediatrics, he had worked at the Perquet Clinic. There he met Dr. Bernard Dattner, an Austrian physician. Dr. Dattner worked with seizure patients, and his theory was that dietary intake could be responsible for the occurrence and severity of the seizures. Leading with this belief, he requested his patients to keep a food journal of everything they consumed and the outcome from this trial appeared to validate his theory. His study did not include synthetic additives because the existence of them in Viennese foods was minimal.

Dr. Feingold also recalled his forty-year-old female patient with hives and her dramatically improved behaviors while on the K-P Diet. What if such a diet would yield the same benefits for children with H-LD? He surmised that little to no deliberation had gone into the connection between food and these patients' hyperactive behavior and decided to make this his next quest. He learned that synthetic flavoring additives were not widely used before World War II, so they were less than thirty-five years old. He discovered a graph with notable similarities between the rising "dollar-value increase" of synthetic flavors, and escalating numbers of reported H-LD cases. Confident that he was moving in the right direction, he became vocal about his discoveries and got the attention of the San Francisco station, KPIX, in October of 1972. During the interview, he shared his theory that synthetic additives in foods could affect H-LD and were somehow, "tampering with the brain and nervous system by short-circuiting some functions in a particular group of children genetically predisposed to these chemicals."

It was from this interview that a mother of a highly energized boy made an appointment with Dr. Feingold. Her son had been under medical care for several years for his disruptive behaviors, and the situation was not improving. The doctor had an EEG done to rule out epilepsy even though he had no evidence of seizure activity. When the test did not show any abnormalities (sometimes these tests are not accurate on hyperkinetic children), the mother was advised to think about family therapy. If that solution did not improve the situation, then medication was the next step. When Dr. Feingold saw the young boy he appeared to be healthy and calm, and the mother explained that she had been following his diet advice from the interview. Since the K-P Diet seemed to be working, Dr. Feingold gave his mother full details regarding implementation. During the trial period, the boy did sneak food a few times, and his personality issues reflected his cheating, and the result was a success.

In examining a child appearing to be hyperactive, Dr. Feingold would use the Descriptive Characteristics of Clinical Pattern of H-LD guide. It is difficult to diagnose this disorder, as each child is different and there are almost a hundred symptoms that characterize hyperactivity. The most common of these are excitability, fidgetiness, aggressive, disruptive, short attention span, compulsive, reckless, impulsiveness, and cries easily. However, there are children with this disorder who do not exhibit these behaviors and are instead unobtrusive, though signs of muscle tone and coordination symptoms are often present. Dr. Feingold generally recommended using the K-P Diet first because he was not a supporter of Ritalin. He believed drugs should be used to treat an ailment only if the benefit outweighed the risk. There needed to be a consideration about the severity and type of illness, the age, weight of the patient, correct dosage, and the presence of any additional medications and chemicals. Dr. Feingold recognized that some physicians believed prescribing appropriate drug therapy with a proper dose could cure an ailment with little to no risk. However, his viewpoint was, "It is now well known that this simplistic concept is fraught with danger."

Only a few studies had been done on the possibility of addiction resulting from drug management. Dr. Feingold stated, "There is ample evidence they can become a psychological crutch. Logic plus medical experience compels me to believe that no patient, particularly no child, can be drug managed for eight years or more, beginning at the age of three or four, without risk. I believe medications should be used only as a last resort when everything else - certainly including the diet - has been tried and failed."

In 1971, the National Health Institute estimated that 300,000 children took amphetamines or Ritalin for hyperactivity (ADHD) and as of 2017, it was determined that 3,721,120 children from age four to seventeen are taking medication. After WWII, there was a concern about drug abuse so the Food and Drug Administration constrained the use of amphetamines for children. Two years later they would reduce the amount of Ritalin that could be manufactured and placed it on the Schedule II List with codeine, morphine, and opium. Yet, in forty-six years, the medical and pharmaceutical communities' best solution has been to place 3,421,120 *more* children on medication. This idea of "progress" is simply unacceptable.

Dr. Feingold noted that a few cases of H-LD children did show improvement on the K-P Diet without their allergies being addressed, but greater success was attained using diet *and* managing the allergies. In one study of twenty-five hyperactive patients on the K-P Diet, seventeen achieved favorable results, showed more self-control, were less distracted, and were easier to manage. There were eight children who did not benefit, but this could be explained by undiagnosed medical conditions, lack of parental cooperation, or the child's failure to adhere to the diet. As Feingold said, "The diet management cannot succeed if parental management is weak or wavering. It is important to recognize that children are not able to make decisions for themselves. Their impulsive behavior is beyond their control."

Feingold felt it was paramount to look more closely at a patient's genetics, environment, and health information to get a better understanding of them. Once he had a clearer picture of a child with H-LD, he presented the K-P Diet to the parents with the expectation that it would be implemented according to the guidelines. He understood how difficult the process would be at first, and harder depending on the child's age, but the reward was worth the effort.

"Most children don't want to be bad," he stated, "on drugs, or in learning-disability classes. They are not sub-intelligent. In my opinion, they are chemically abused. These children are normal. Their environment is abnormal."

The first manufactured coal-tar color used in food was mauve and created by Sir William Henry Perkins in 1856. In just forty-four years, around eighty coal-tar colors were being used in foods and clothing. It was Dr. Henry Washington Wiley who raised the first alarm about the use of these colors. As the chief chemist with the Department of Agriculture, he knew the potential threat from these dyes and stated, "The American people are steadily poisoned by dangerous chemicals added to food with reckless abandon." Six years later, finally acting upon his warning, a "Food and Drug Act" was presented to Congress and then to President Theodore Roosevelt for his signature. Within a year of the creation of the FDA, all but seven of the synthetic colors were prohibited. By 1973, of those seven colors that were allowed, four were later found to be inherently harmful and eliminated. To date, there are eight artificial colors approved by the FDA in food.

Synthetic flavorings were also being used in foods, with twenty-six on the Generally Recognized as Safe (GRAS) list, as well as an estimated 1,500 other flavors within the "flavor enhancing" category. Today, there are 700 such flavors on the GRAS list, with an estimated 2,000 other flavors being used as enhancers or modifiers. Dr. Feingold did not waver in his concern that though they were regarded as safe, they still could, "possibly be disrupting the normal neurological pathways of the nervous system."

Dr. Bert N. LaDu weighed in with his concerns about the rise of synthetics: "A person has his own biological individuality that determines a pharmacological individuality." In simpler terms, each person has a unique DNA; some will be able to tolerate certain chemicals while others will not be able to tolerate them.

In May of 1974, a case study was done on children assigned to a care facility in Redwood Valley, California, for severe issues with behavior. They ranged in age from three to seventeen and had been diagnosed with such conditions as Autism, neurological disorders, emotional disorders, behavioral disorders and/or learning disabilities. All eleven children were placed on the K-P Diet with no ability to deviate from the restriction. Within two weeks, there was a noticeable difference in the behaviors of the children: six of them showed improvement; two had a slight change; and the three remaining had no change, but two of them had autism.

These impressive results showed the effectiveness of following the K-P Diet with no opportunity to cheat. In Dr. Feingold's first study of the K-P Diet on twenty-five of his patients, he learned that "Along with the successes, there have been partial to complete failures with eight not responding to the K-P Diet. The same ratio, more or less, has continued as experience broadens. The best estimate is that fifty percent have a likelihood of full response, while seventy-five percent can be removed from drug management." In Rebecca's case, I tried to simplify things by having her tested for food allergies before starting the K-P Diet. Although she showed no signs of food allergies, she did have an intolerance to natural foods that are orange in color. It was using the food diary that helped me discover this information.

The third study on the K-P Diet was funded by the Department of Education of Santa Cruz, California. Twenty-five students, some of whom were on medication, served as the test group. Other participants included a psychologist, teachers already working with the children, a nutritionist, and cooperating parents. Of the twenty-five students, twelve showed an improvement, nine did not change, and four failed to follow the diet. These studies were beneficial, but Dr. Feingold wanted a study to be done on some children at the Kaiser Permanente Pediatrics Department. He wanted a pediatrician to examine them and have a nurse practitioner work closely with the parents on implementing the K-P Diet. All ten children had successful results, and four were able to stop their medication.

I can personally attest that adhering strictly to the guidelines of the K-P Diet brought about drastic and positive changes in Rebecca's behavior. Once her body was clean, she told me that she felt "different" inside, which is most likely why she was good at avoiding unsafe foods. Dr. Feingold thought it essential to understand that, "Children who react to the synthetic additives have genetic variations – not abnormalities - which predispose them to such adverse responses. It is not the child's fault, nor are the parents responsible for this quirk of nature." The mass production of synthetics made packaged food more appealing and last longer and little consideration was given to the possibility that the chemicals had the potential to impact the pathways neurologically for everyone, not just those who have ADHD.

Dr. Feingold could not help but hypothesize that these chemicals were "possibly disrupting the normal neurological pathways of the nervous system."

As two-time Nobel Prize winner Dr. Linus Pauling stated, "Psychiatry predicated upon the interaction of chemicals and the homeostasis, or balance, of chemicals in the body. All the human psychological processes are dependent upon the proper balance, the concentration of various chemicals inside the cells and outside of them. If an imbalance occurs, a malfunction may develop."

Expanding on Pauling's theory, Dr. Feingold indicated that, "Insanity is a disease of the brain, not a matter of intellect. No one knows why the imbalance takes place, nor how it works, but medical science is slowly groping toward an answer. It would appear vitally necessary to examine both natural and synthetic chemicals in our food and learn how they interrelate."

I will be forever grateful to Dr. Benjamin F. Feingold for his life's work and his decision to postpone his retirement to help children affected by ADHD. He passed away in 1982, but his awe-inspiring devotion to his patients' lives on through his research and writings. His K-P Diet drastically changed our lives, along with countless others. I am so thankful that I decided to take the road less traveled with regard to treatment because it literally saved Rebecca's childhood, and without the use of dangerous medications.

CHAPTER FIVE

Learning to use the Feingold Diet

"The most difficult thing is the decision to act, the rest is merely tenacity. The fears are paper tigers. You can do anything you decide to do."

Amelia Earhart

Sheryl was successful in convincing the administrators of the DLC to give Rebecca another chance and me a month in which to incorporate the K-P Diet into her daily regimen. Though Sheryl never shared how much adversity she faced while trying to get Rebecca back into class, I knew I owed her a tremendous favor. We had undoubtedly won the lotto where teachers were concerned because Sheryl was an outstanding, caring, and an exceptionally dedicated woman. Without her belief and support, as well as the support of the DLC, I truly believe I would have suffered a mental breakdown. Now, I faced an enormous pressure to prove their support was well-placed and that the new diet would correct Rebecca's defiance.

Reading Dr. Feingold's book had been the lifeline I was searching for and the more I read, the more I felt like he had a window inside Rebecca's body. He dispelled numerous myths I had naively believed and gave me specifics about the complexity of ADHD. I discovered that there were actually two disorders under the ADHD umbrella: Attention Deficit Disorder (ADD), which does not include hyperactivity, and Attention Deficit Hyperactivity Disorder (ADHD), which does include it. The consensus was that while both disorders are believed to be genetic, they are not "diseases." There are also various aspects of the disorders that are sometimes associated with Learning Disabilities (LD).

It was encouraging to read the documentation on children who responded well to the diet, and I was optimistic that this course would manage Rebecca's hyperactivity. Of course there were moments when I wondered whether I was grasping at straws in order to avoid medication; however, my instincts kept telling me that this safe and natural method was the best option for my daughter. In fact, once I knew the potential dangers attached to Ritalin (a stimulant), Dexedrine (an amphetamine), and Stelazine (a tranquilizer), I was more determined than ever to do whatever it took to spare Rebecca from them.

Both Ritalin and Dexedrine were on the FDA's Schedule II Controlled Substance List due to the potential for abuse and possibly psychological or physical dependence. I also asked a physician if it was true that there was a possibility of an additional drug becoming necessary after extended use of Ritalin. His reply - "Apparently, you have done your homework" – was just further confirmation that I had made the right decision.

That does not mean I didn't fear failure; however, as I had done throughout my life, I channeled that fear into commitment and *expected* that my hard work would lead to victory. First, I needed to create a game plan, namely, that this would be a family affair. All of us, not just Rebecca, would embrace the all-natural diet. I was not too worried about Rebecca being agreeable to the change because she was still young enough to trust me with her care. My opposition would be in trying to convince Greg and Stephanie and impress upon them that this route was an alternative to pills. Realistically, I knew my only chance to sell this proposal was to provide them with an option of cheating "offsite." The three of us would eat whatever we wanted away from Rebecca, but in her presence we all ate the new-fangled way.

When I was explaining things to Greg, he gave me that look over his glasses, which meant he was perplexed about the words coming out of my mouth. Stephanie was agreeable to trying if there was a possibility that it would change Rebecca's unruly behavior. That's the thing about living in a war zone: folks are more approachable when presented with a hair-brained idea because they are tired of being powerless and desire an improvement. As for me, I approached this challenge with the mindset that I had little to lose and so very much to gain.

My next obstacle was to explain the diet to Rebecca. I kept it simple, telling her that the doctor said eating this new way would make her feel calmer and have fewer tantrums. I also told her that I, her father and Stephanie would be eating it as well, which was sure to bring about greater cooperation than if she was going it alone. The only thing I didn't mention was that the "doctor" I spoke of was not our physician, but Dr. Feingold.

I made sure that Rebecca understood that once the diet began, she could not eat anything unless it was checked first by me to make sure it was safe and would not make her sick. By repeatedly using the word "sick" I helped her make the connection between what she ate and its potential effect on her body. Again, Rebecca was four years old with no reason not to trust that I had her best interests at heart. She accepted the new rules and promised to follow them, which made things much more convenient. Now it was time to focus on meal prep and the reality that many things would require cooking and baking the old-fashioned way, as in *from scratch*. Thus I said goodbye to one of the few stress-free aspects of my life: mealtimes. Like many busy parents, I had relied on an abundance of prepackaged foods and the wonderful invention of the microwave. Heck, I could come racing in the back door and throw something in a pan or on a cookie sheet and have dinner on the table in thirty minutes or less!

It took some time and effort to get the diet formulated, and I reminded myself that this hurdle was for my family and they were worth the effort. Besides, it did not take a rocket scientist to figure out it was healthier to eat natural foods than the stuff that came in boxes and cans and were loaded with chemicals and dyes. Well, to be honest, I did not think about it much until after reading Dr. Feingold's book, and yes, there was plenty of whining being done as I went through the cupboards removing all but the natural foods. This was the first time I had paid any attention to the foods we were eating and dismayed to realize how much of our diet revolved around so many unhealthy fast and ready-to-eat products. Now, as I tossed cookies, chips, Tuna Helper, Hamburger Helper, canned soups, cereals, bread, jellies, and candy onto the kitchen table to be donated to my family (actually, the candy went into the drawer of my nightstand so I could appease the sweet tooth inherited from my mom), the little cash register in my mind was going "cha-ching" for all the money that was being wasted.

Needless to say, I was not overly enthusiastic at this point and I had only begun tackling the trials and tribulations that this undertaking was going to entail. To bolster my determination, I gave myself the pep talk about how the first step in any venture is always the most difficult and that I just needed to focus on taking it one day at a time. I followed Creighton Abrams Jr.'s words of wisdom in facing this challenge: "When eating an elephant take one bite at a time." This quote has resonated with me throughout my life and always helps remind me that any situation is manageable if it is broken into easy steps. To prevent being overwhelmed, I had to pace myself and trust my Irish intuition that it would become simpler in time. It was as if someone was dangling the proverbial carrot with the stick in front of me, except in my case the carrot was a yummy chocolate bar.

Next, I had to remove all foods with natural salicylates in all their forms. These include almonds, apples, apricots, blackberries, boysenberries, gooseberries, raspberries, strawberries, cherries, currants, grapes, raisins and anything else made from grapes, nectarines, oranges, peaches, and prunes. There were also some vegetables on the list, including tomatoes and all products made from them, cucumbers, and pickles. As mentioned before, any processed foods, including meats, baked goods, many kinds of cereal, chips, and beverages, were prohibited as well. (If you are reading this and feel overwhelmed, trust me, it does get easier and is only a temporary inconvenience for a positive lifelong outcome. You can do this!)

And those were just the foods. Since we absorb things through our skin, I also had to check the labels on the soap, shampoo, toothpaste, lotions, et cetera., to make sure they were natural and free of artificial colors, dyes, or preservatives. This is where the importance of keeping a daily diary comes in. To be successfully, you *must* write every food your child eats and what they drink and how they behave after. Charting was the principal component that helped me spot problem behaviors directly linked to something Rebecca ingested. This record is also beneficial in determining what food and beverages your child can tolerate and which ones to remove due to an intolerance. Every child is different, but you should see a positive change in your child's behavior in about three to six weeks.

The third invaluable step is having a behavior modification plan in place when you begin the food elimination process. Though many of your child's behavioral problems may be related to the foods they ingest, they are also learned behaviors and therefore can be corrected by instituting a consistent plan. Once you have a handle on the behavioral issues and see improvements using the diet, then you can test a food by adding their favorite one back into their diet. If your child immediately goes off the spool, this is your indication that their body has an intolerance to that food. Just keep adding one new food every four days and chart their behavior; if it is good, then that is another food item that is safe for your child. I know it sounds daunting, but it really is a key step and the only way to test for a reaction to specific foods.

By utilizing this test method, I discovered that although the allergy tests administered by our doctor came back negative for food allergies,

Rebecca did in fact have an intolerance to oranges, carrots, and yellow cheese; she also required three days in between having ketchup. If someone has an intolerance to certain foods, they may develop a rash or show a change in behavior, and it generally takes up to seventy-two hours for the body to recover from the reaction. That is why keeping a food and behavior diary is an essential tool for you to become a food detective. The key components of using the Feingold Diet to manage Rebecca's unruly behavior successfully required absolute commitment and consistency.

Cleaning out the cupboards turned out to be a relatively painless task compared to grocery shopping. Today, you can go into nearly any supermarket and find an endless supply of healthy food choices including organic, dairy-free and gluten-free, as well as other products free of chemicals, artificial colors, flavors and preservatives. Back then, natural foods were slim to none and reading the list of ingredients on the labels was like trying to learn a foreign language. Since most prepackaged foods were no longer an option, I left the store that first time with only a few fresh fruits, vegetables, and some cheese. Clearly another trip to the library was in order, this time so I could educate myself about food additives. I put together a list of artificial additives, preservatives, and colors, and this became my cheat sheet when I returned for round two at the grocery store. Now, I had a starting point for what was considered artificial and so was able to purchase more items. This process made it more straightforward and less frustrating.

The first morning of the diet, Rebecca was not happy about giving up her orange juice and pouted a little, but thankfully, the battle was relatively minor. Surprisingly, Rebecca was dedicated to this new way of eating and did not cheat, which was awesome. Going to restaurants was difficult because I could not ensure the food was safe, but once I explained our situation to the servers, they did what they could to help. There was also communication with the kitchen for accurate information on how to avoid cross-contamination. Rebecca would mostly order a plain hamburger without a bun, condiments, or seasonings, and the

French fires were without seasonings as well. We also ate home more, which was a benefit to our budget.

Meal planning was not something that I regularly did, so it was a struggle to sit down and plan a daily menu. My shopping style at the grocery store was to toss items we liked into the cart, then I would get creative making different meals from the packages and cans. Now that I was no longer able to fly by the seat of my pants, I finally put my Betty Crocker Cookbook - that wedding gift from my mom - to good use. I loved baking so that part was not too difficult, and I soon realized that most of the meals were easy to fix with fresh meats and veggies. Overall, the journey on this new way of shopping and eating was slightly more time consuming but honestly not as overwhelming as it had initially seemed.

Rebecca responded favorably to all the changes, and the number of reprimands for her negative behavior began to decrease. Within a couple of weeks, there was a drastic reduction in her excessive movements and fewer temper tantrums. She was not as calm and compliant as her sister, but she was definitely less manic than before starting the diet. We were elated with her progress, and I once again kicked my butt for not reading Dr. Feingold's book the day Mom gave it to me. So many situations and frustrations could have been avoided if I had been smarter!

About a month into the diet, I decided to introduce one food back into her diet. I chose a Friday night to do this because if she had a food reaction it would take seventy-two hours before her body was clean and calm again. When Rebecca did have a negative response, she described the feeling as, "My brain feels like it is buzzing and my head hurts." She was not as aggressive as before and though there was still a bit of a temper, she was responding well to discipline.

Again, I want to impress how important the food diary is for your insight into what is and is not working. Life can be very hectic, so charting foods and behaviors will help you discover the difference between a busy day and a possible food reaction. A few times, I wondered why Rebecca seemed to be out of sorts when no new food item had been introduced, and it was by looking at the diary that I was able to discover what caused the unrest. One time it was because she had ingested ketchup without the three-day waiting period that she needed in order to be able to tolerate it.

Two months later, Sheryl wrote the following progress report: "Rebecca is making good progress on her goals and her behavior improvement from the diet is remarkable. She initiates play with other students, asks for things before taking them, and is doing a wonderful job."

The change in Rebecca's behavior was accomplished solely by changing her diet and consistently using the behavior management techniques already implemented. This drastic improvement, along with help from our hero, Sheryl, had saved Rebecca from being expelled from the DLC.

Class time was now a learning environment rather than Rebecca's battlefield, and Sheryl and her aides made a difference by helping to monitor what Rebecca was exposed to in the classroom. I packed her lunch each day, provided all her snacks, and was genuinely fortunate that Rebecca was so terrific about not eating food or treats offered to her from the other children. We were extremely proud of her for the excellent job she did in maintaining her diet. I believe her greatest incentive to keep her body clean was that she could not tolerate the "brain buzzing and terrible headaches." My purse became a walking snack bag wherever we went to ensure that I always had something for Rebecca to eat. When we were invited to someone's house for dinner, I prepared her meal at home and brought it along with us. Once people understood Rebecca had an intolerance to certain foods and drinks, they were extremely accommodating. We continued using the word, "safe for you" to remind Rebecca that her health was more important than any food or treat that she wanted.

When a child is in Special Education classes, an Individual Education Plan (IEP) is created for them to set educational goals. Administrators also schedule an Individual Education Plan (IEP) meeting to discuss with parents these goals and the progress their son or daughter is making toward achieving them. During Rebecca's IEP meeting at the

DLC, the supervising staff member commented after reviewing the latest evaluation that she would not have believed this was the same child. This woman knew that Rebecca was being expelled for severe behavioral problems and found it hard to believe that food changes had made the difference. Not that I needed validation for choosing an alternative to medication, but her statement was uplifting to my confidence.

I would estimate that it took our family about two months to become accustomed to eating the Feingold way. By this time Rebecca had become so comfortable with the diet that we felt comfortable eating foods she could not so long as she had similar foods items. Then, just when I thought we had it down, I began encountering several obstacles. I had not thought ahead to hurdles like birthday parties at school, Valentine's Day, Easter Baskets, and Halloween. These were just some of life's events that for most children were simply fun but had the potential to derail the progress we had made.

You know the saying it takes a village to raise a child? Well, that sure as heck is accurate in the case of an ADHD and Special Needs child. It is imperative on the first day of school to communicate with your child's teacher and share insight into his or her needs. This includes any food intolerances, the behavioral program you are using, and a desire to have open communication so you always know how things are going in the classroom. Since many children with ADHD also have learning disabilities and medical issues, it truly does take a team to help them achieve academic success. Realistically, even without medical or mental problems, teachers never could adequately educate the children without the input and involvement of the parents.

Thankfully, the teachers were very good at explaining to her classmates that Rebecca had food allergies and they should never give her anything to eat. There were several occasions when compassionate classmates brought Rebecca an apple when they had birthday treats for the class. I did provide snacks to keep on hand in the classroom for such situations, but it was remarkable that several classmates wanted to include her with bringing the apples.

There was one exception early on. It was Rebecca's first Valentine Day's party at school and she came home all ramped up with excitement with her bag of goodies. When I asked her to empty the sack so we could separate the candy from the Valentine's she refused, a new behavior. She had not fought me before about giving up something she could not eat in exchange for something safe. When I attempted to reach for the bag, she took a swing at me, so I forcibly removed the bag, which provoked screaming and crying. Rebecca tried to grab the sack out of my hand, and I sent her upstairs to her bedroom. Once she had settled down, I asked why she had acted like that when she knew that she could not eat the candy. She explained that it was her first Valentine's and wanted to go through it herself and had planned on giving the candy to her dad and sister. I apologized to her for not thinking it through in my haste to remove the candy. Lesson learned!

I asked her how we could make the situation better, and she suggested I take her to Target for a five-dollar toy to replace her goody bag. I realized then that this was a better exchange than goodies from the cupboard on special occasions like Easter, Halloween, and Christmas. Before the diet, I took the girls over to my parents' house to Trick or Treat at the same houses I had frequented as a child. There was one older man who always made you perform a trick for your treat, and he was still at it when I took Stephanie and Rebecca. Of course, when he asked Rebecca to show him a trick if she wanted the candy, she told him to forget it. He was so tickled by this he gave her double the candy. Heck, I wish I had been smart enough to think of that reply when I was a kid.

Now thinking ahead, it seemed cruel to have her collect a bag of candy and then take it away, so I created a unique Halloween tradition. Before I presented the idea to the girls, I took Stephanie aside, explained my plan and told her it was okay if she chose to go out with her friends. Instead, that incredibly compassionate daughter of mine decided to stay home so Rebecca would not be alone. God sure picked a great big sister for Rebecca! Stephanie pretended to be hearing my plan for the first time as I explained that they would still go to Target to pick out costumes and get five dollars to buy whatever they wanted, but we would be staying home to hand out candy and watch the movie ET. The girls enjoyed giving out candy but decided that they wanted to go out trick-or-treating the next year. When Halloween rolled around once again, I had mixed emotions about it, given the drama of Rebecca's first Valentine's party. On the other hand, I also knew I needed to be selective about what limitations I presented. The last thing I wanted was to have Rebecca become resentful of the diet. So, before I consented, she had to agree that the candy was not the prize. Thankfully, she was already a step ahead and more than happy to give up her loot for a trip to Target.

Rebecca was still making progress at the DLC when the regular school district began testing for kindergarten. Wanting to have her evaluated but wary of hearing the reservations from the supervisors at the DLC, I refrained from discussing the subject with them. Out of respect for Sheryl, I did give her a heads-up of my compelling desire to know precisely what Rebecca's capabilities were beyond the Special Education environment. None of us knew what Rebecca was capable of learning as we pushed her until she got frustrated and started to shut down. We needed this opportunity to discover if Rebecca had made sufficient progress to make it in a regular classroom environment. Sheryl agreed that the testing could be valuable in assessing Rebecca's abilities, so I took her to the appointment. We were surprised and ecstatic when the notification came that Rebecca had met the requirements to enter the regular kindergarten class.

Whenever one embarks on a life-changing program or process, there will be times when it feels like there are more struggles than successes. That had certainly been the case in the first year we implemented the diet. Now, to receive objective confirmation of her progress was simply amazing. When I shared the good news with her, Sheryl was both happy for Rebecca and sad because she had enjoyed having her in class (this, considering her history, was in and of itself an incredible thing to hear). Now, the next step was to meet with the supervisors of the DLC for what's referred to as the "Trial-Out."

As we began this process, Greg and I were surprised to find that it was more involved than we imagined. First, we needed *permission* to take Rebecca out of the DLC. In our desperation we had missed this important detail in the fine print, that in accepting their help we were signing away some of our decision-making power as Rebecca's parents. Another valuable lesson learned! Second, when we presented our formal request to remove Rebecca, they honored our request but with a significant stipulation: their approval was temporary pending an evaluation from the kindergarten teacher at the end of the first quarter. We were shocked they had that much control in our lives and had to remind ourselves that without them we would not have made it to this very encouraging juncture in our journey.

Though we were excited to take this next step it would be difficult to say goodbye to Sheryl, who was not only Rebecca's teacher but our friend, mentor, cheerleader, and advocate. That last day was certainly bittersweet, but our sadness was mitigated by the knowledge that we would see her again. Sheryl was getting married that summer and had asked Rebecca to be her flower girl! Of course, I was honored, and Rebecca was ecstatic about being in the wedding and that her best school buddy was to serve as ring bearer.

It was a beautiful wedding. The bride was radiant, and the flower girl did a fantastic job, looking so darn angelic as she walked down the aisle and danced into the night. It was an excellent way to end a chapter in our lives that had given us so many blessings. Sheryl had set the bar very high, in my opinion, at the caliber of teacher we could expect and I prayed diligently that the kindergarten teacher would be as dedicated as she. Unfair perhaps, but when you start at the top anything less is bound to be frustrating and challenging.

Over the summer break it was my responsibility to keep working academically with Rebecca. From Margo I had learned the necessity of keeping Rebecca learning regardless of the seasons because her brain deficit affected her memory. To keep her from losing what she had learned and knowing structure was important, I created a "classroom" that Rebecca attended each morning during the week. After breakfast, Rebecca would go to play until mid-morning, then come to sit at the kitchen table and work. I had created worksheets from the papers she brought home from school throughout the year. We called this endeavor our summertime fun class. We started with coloring to get her relaxed, and then I maneuvered her attention toward projects for which she had to sit still and stay focused. To keep her from fighting this process, I kept the sessions to just about an hour - a bit longer if it was raining - and then she was free to play the rest of the day.

Most days, Rebecca was cooperative during our academic hour. On the few occasions when she fought against my homeschooling system, I brought out the button jar so we could sort by color and size and then count them. She was unaware that this fun strategy was working on her ability to sit still and stay on task. The presentation of the information was not as important as how long I had her work, because if I frustrated her she would just shut down and refuse to budge. This presented a challenge to me to be creative and keep learning fun, and thankfully, Stephanie and her friends often came to my aid, joining in on the coloring, puzzles, reading, counting, painting, and drawing to keep Rebecca busy.

As always, when things grew trying I focused on my goal: preventing her first day of kindergarten from becoming a repeat of her first day of preschool, with a negative phone call from the teacher. It was in everyone's best interest that I remained diligent at keeping Rebecca accustomed to a structured learning environment with the expectations of required behavior within the classroom. Most parents probably never worry much about a new school year beginning because the year before was without mishaps. Our experiences had been vastly different, and although we had made significant progress with the diet and behavior, it was Rebecca's learning deficits and personality traits that always seemed to cause duress. These two problems continued to stress and worry me about her starting kindergarten. It was very much like standing on the edge of a dock watching Rebecca jump in without a life vest and me holding my breath waiting to see if she would sink or swim.

CHAPTER SIX

The Launching of Kindergarten

"Take the first step in faith. You don't have to see the whole staircase. Just take the first step."

Martin Luther King, Jr.

The first day of kindergarten finally arrived. Despite my trepidations, my heart was singing with joy as I picked out her prettiest dress and the white vinyl dress shoes for this very monumental moment in her life. She may not have been aware of the significance of that first day, but I was. Since she would be attending the afternoon class, I made sure that her morning routine was calm and relaxed so she would not be in her supercharge mode. Butler School was about three blocks away, so we walked there, and when we arrived at her classroom, I introduced myself to her teacher. Elizabeth was very polite, and her sincere greeting gave me great vibes, which went a long way to easing my worries.

Elizabeth expressed that she was comfortable following the request of the DLC and using their skill's checklist to record and measure Rebecca's growth. We then chatted about the diet. I gave her snacks for Rebecca and asked her to ensure that the children knew not to give her anything to eat. Elizabeth seemed undaunted by all the special requests being made of her and truly supportive about having Rebecca in her classroom. She assured me her policy was to use a firm, yet gentle manner with all her students and that she was confident it would be just fine. This type of optimism was unlike our previous first day experiences that on my walk home I decided it was too good to be true. I just knew that before the day was over that dreaded phone call would come and confirm that I was in fact delusional.

Rebecca came home from school excited about her first day. I continued to wait for the phone to ring and was shocked when it didn't. Although I was relieved, my radar was still programmed to be in the hypervigilant mode of waiting for the other shoe to drop. However, as the days went on, Rebecca was happy, content, and doing well at school, and the other children respected the fact that she was on a special diet and didn't give her anything to eat. So far, Rebecca's journey into the standard academic world was more than I had thought possible, and for the first time I believed that I might be able to let go of my apprehension. After years of being both on high alert and emotionally drained, this new experience was liberating. It was like getting permission to relax, let my guard down, and embrace the belief that we had jumped our last hurdle.

Elizabeth was excellent at implementing open communication so that I could monitor Rebecca's behavior and progress within the classroom. Things continued to be inspiring, and it reinforced our conviction that Greg and I had made the right decision in having her tested. On the DLC's quarterly progress report, Elizabeth had written, "Rebecca is responding well to a firm approach regarding discipline and following directions. Overall, she seems to understand the concepts taught and is behaving appropriately in the classroom. Rebecca has developed the skills expected of kindergarten students at this time and is continuing to develop some independent work skills."

My feet were barely touching the ground when I read that report! Greg was equally overjoyed and we savored this accomplishment and anticipated continued success. Then the letter arrived from the DLC informing us that our attendance was required at a meeting they had scheduled.

My first reaction was negative since I was still irritated that they oversaw our daughter's education, and I had to prepare myself for the meeting mentally. They surprised me with their statement that Rebecca had shown enough success learning the letters of the alphabet, as well as their sounds, and appeared to be learning the information presented. She had developed the necessary skills required for kindergarten, and they deemed her ready to be staffed out of the Special Education Program, with one stipulation. A specialist was working with Rebecca on her Speech and Language skills, and that service would continue.

Though I wasn't thrilled that the DLC would continue to have a foothold in our lives, I embraced having another fantastic teacher who was dedicated to helping Rebecca reach her potential. As the saying goes, count your blessings! You know that other saying, "Life happens when you are busy making other plans?" Well, it would seem life thought I was getting just too comfortable, because shortly after that meeting Rebecca came home after school exhibiting signs of a food reaction. I knew I had not introduced anything new, and Elizabeth was vigilant about monitoring the classroom, so I suspected Rebecca had ingested something outside of class. I asked her if she had accepted something to eat from a child during recess, but she was adamant that she had not.

At a loss as to what was going on, I took Rebecca to class the next day and told Elizabeth that she was displaying signs of a food reaction. I explained that the cause mystified me and asked if she had any ideas, but she reassured me that the other children had been excellent about not giving her food or candy. Despite her confidence, I was concerned about letting Rebecca stay for the class, for fear that she would exhibit her old behaviors. Undaunted, Elizabeth promised to have the office call if there were any problems. Though my mind was screaming, "Please no, not the office!" I conceded and left Rebecca there. Thank goodness there was no phone call before I returned to picked her up, however when I asked

Elizabeth if there had been any issues, she declared that while Rebecca had looked like her usual sweet little self, her attitude and the energy were definitely not the child she knew.

She then shared that a few times she had needed to reprimand Rebecca in order to keep her on task but felt it was not drastic enough to call me. She then mentioned that several days before she had brought carrots to school for snacks, and since they were natural, felt it was safe to give one to Rebecca. I now had the answer to what had caused the food reaction, and it was my fault! When I had explained the diet to her, I had failed to mention that she also had an intolerance to some *natural* foods and drinks as well, including oranges, yellow cheeses…and carrots. Another lesson learned. I apologized to Elizabeth and made a mental note that the next time I told someone new about the diet I had to make it clear that artificial ingredients were not the only culprits.

Aside from that mishap the schoolyear was relatively calm, and for the first time we had made it through without a call from school or a negative report from the teacher. We were brimming with pride for Rebecca and felt her hard work and diligence had absolutely earned her a big celebration and a trip to Target. She was enthusiastic about school being over and looking forward to the fun of summer, but just as before, I structured in some learning activities. At midday, Monday through Friday, we were sitting at the kitchen table working on her academics so she would be ready for first grade.

As it turned out, the transition from kindergarten to first grade would not be as smooth. Sheryl and Elizabeth had taught me that working with a teacher is not only optimal but necessary to cultivate a successful learning environment for Rebecca; however, this new teacher appeared rather indifferent to my wanting to share Rebecca's history or my request for open communication. In fact I got the distinct impression that she was in charge and not interested in my insight regarding how Rebecca learned best. Just as I expected, within several weeks, Rebecca was struggling to maintain the academic level expected. I reached out to the teacher and requested a meeting, hoping she would be open to collaboration.

However, it only took a few minutes of that meeting for me to realize that I could expect discord from her, rather than unity.

Never had my strategic suggestions regarding Rebecca been shot down, one after the other, by a teacher. She expected all her students to function the same and did not have the time or the willingness to offer any additional assistance. This teacher had a firm sink or swim mentality for all the children in her classroom, and in my opinion, she commanded rather than taught. Feeling as though she'd left me without an option, I went to speak with the principal who had not been quick enough to leave the building. He was polite and gave me a few minutes of his time in which to share my concerns regarding this teacher; clearly, we had a personality conflict that was going to make working together impossible. As I spoke, I was reasonably optimistic that he would move Rebecca into the other first-grade classroom. Problem solved, right? Wrong. After expressing his extreme confidence in this teacher's abilities, he promptly denied my request. I had been dismissed.

Well, the writing was on the wall as they say, and I knew this was going to be a horrible school year, and there was nothing more I could do to avoid the outcome. Even though I worked diligently with Rebecca at home to help her comprehend her homework assignments, I was unable to support her in the classroom, where she desperately needed the assistance. The situation was incredibly frustrating for Rebecca, and I was powerless to make it better. It was discouraging and exasperating to have a teacher who did not impart the same caliber of enthusiasm for teaching as Sheryl and Elizabeth. They were devoted professionals striving to make sure that their students understood what they were teaching and encouraged me to be part of the team. Their jobs were made easier, and Rebecca's successes were much grander, because of the joint effort.

Rebecca also started acting out at school, the first time on the playground during recess and the second time during lunch. One day she was on the slide and getting ready to go down when a boy pushed her from behind. Thankfully, she managed to stay on the slide, though her body was not lined up correctly. The ride down was scary, bumpy, and far from gentle as she flew off and landed on her butt. She got to her feet ready for battle and my little hellcat, much like her momma, was waiting for the boy when he came down the slide laughing. She gave him one good punch that sent him crying into school, which resulted in a call home to inform me that Rebecca had struck another child. When I asked what had prompted this altercation, I was told there was no reason. Her punishment therefore was to remain inside for the remainder of recess.

When Rebecca came home, I asked for her version of what happened. She told me about being pushed and that she was defending herself. I asked if the teacher had asked for her side of the story, and she said, "Nope." As Rebecca has always been an extremely honest child, I did not question her account for a minute. I did remind her, however, of "Papa's Rule," which had been taught to me by my dad when I was about Rebecca's age. My siblings and I were raised to be peaceful and never allowed to throw the first punch, but if someone hit us, then we certainly had permission to defend ourselves. Though the boy had shoved her, Rebecca had broken the rule. Since she had already been punished at school, I just gave her a timeout. The next morning before she left for school, I asked how she was going to handle problems.

"With my words, Mom," she replied, "and not with my hands."

Unfortunately, that theory is for folks with tempers that are slow to ignite, and Rebecca still struggled with a short fuse, which meant it would just be a matter of time before it happened again.

We barely made it a month before the next phone call, and the secretary was informing me that Rebecca had knocked two girls' heads together at lunch and would be losing recess privileges again, this time for a few days. When I inquired as to what these girls had said or done to cause Rebecca to react that way, she replied that the girls reported doing nothing to Rebecca. Then I asked her what Rebecca had to say about the situation and apparently, Rebecca said, "They were bugging me, so I shut them up, end of story." Of course, I understood how the school would have a problem with that answer, but it irritated me that they so readily believed Rebecca was in the wrong. I grew up with the logic that it takes two to tangle, so I expressed my thoughts that perhaps the girls had said something to antagonize Rebecca. The woman countered that the girls did not provoke the altercation and were the victims since Rebecca had stood up and assaulted them. It was the same as when I had spoken to the principal and after the slide incident: a unilateral determination made by the school - no further discussion, case closed.

I was waiting for Rebecca when she got home from school. When I asked for her side of the story, she said that for the last couple of days these girls had taunted her from across the lunch table. She had tried to do as I told her and use her words and tell them to stop, but they would not listen. Finally she got fed up, knocked their heads together, then sat down to finish her lunch. In her mind, she was justified in her action because she had used her words several times and they failed to stop. Of course once again, she had forgotten the part about not striking first. Part of me wanted to congratulate her for defending herself from bullies, but being a responsible parent, I did not have that luxury. Instead, she got another lecture and told that regardless of what those girls said or did, she could not hit anyone unless they hit her first. That time I took away a privilege and gave a timeout for not getting the concept about the hitting.

The Luck of the Irish held strong as Rebecca barely squeaked by and passed first grade. By that time she was so frustrated and despised anything to do with school, which made her more stubborn about doing her summer lessons. I needed to step up my game and be creative in my techniques. To keep her mind active and learning, we played games, did a word search for rewards, counted cracks in the sidewalk during walks, and indulged in extra story time before bedtime. Summer seemed to be racing by quickly, and we both dreaded her having to return for second grade. I was determined to make each day as enjoyable as possible, and our favorite activity was walking six blocks to the park and directly over to the mini animal zoo. We would stick pieces of bread through the fence to entice the turkey, donkey, goat, miniature horse, numerous ducks, rabbits, and deer to come over. Once the food was gone, the girls played on the equipment until it was time to put down the blanket for our picnic lunch.

The picnics at the park were the highlight of our summer, and we tried to go as often as possible. One day we had just walked in the door after one of these outings when the phone started ringing. Oh, what a pleasurable sound in the summer compared to when school was in session! It was a nurse from the doctor's office saying Greg's test results had come in, and we needed to make a follow-up appointment. Greg had been bothered for several years with pain in his left knee and finally decided to see an orthopedist, as he was worried that it would begin to affect his job performance. Our hometown had a medical clinic and hospital but limited physicians in specialty medicine, so it was standard procedure to go to a larger town, which is what Greg did. On the day of his appointment, we had with us not only our two girls but my niece, Cassie, who was just a few months old. In addition to my waitressing job, I also provided childcare for several of my nieces and nephews during the week.

It was a beautiful sunny morning, and as we made the ninety-mile trip to Des Moines the girls kept themselves entertained by pretending we were on some grand adventure while Cassie, thankfully, slept most of the way. As we walked into the facility, Rebecca was instantly attracted to the multiple selections of toys and went off to play while Greg checked in. His name was called after a short wait, and I stood with a sleeping Cassie in my arms and reminded Rebecca that Stephanie was in charge. We rarely had issues with her behavior at this point, and she listened well to her sister, so we were not worried about leaving them in the waiting area for what we assumed would be an in and out appointment. We followed the nurse to an exam room where Greg sat down, and I walked over to the window and was swaying with Cassie.

A few minutes later, the doctor entered and introduced himself to me since I had not been with Greg on the first visit. He asked if I wanted to sit down, which I politely declined, thinking nothing good comes from being asked to sit down. Sure enough, the doctor sat across from Greg and told him that the test showed something different from what he had anticipated – there was a cancerous tumor in his knee and the odds were not very good. As I struggled to breathe, the doctor said that though it was a slow-growing cancer it was usually terminal, but Greg was fortunate. Our doctor had just attended a medical conference where a surgeon specializing in this type of cancer was present. Since he had Greg's test results before the meeting, he had taken it upon himself to persuade the surgeon to take Greg's case; this, he felt, increased Greg's chance of survival. The surgeon worked out of the Mayo Clinic in Rochester, Minnesota, which was one of if not the best hospitals in the country. It was also only one hundred eighty-four miles away.

There was nothing more the doctor could do for us, so he told us to take some time to process the news. He then exited the room, leaving me and my husband to sit in shocked silence. All these years, we had believed the pain was due to an old injury from playing sports in school! Greg was only 34 years old, and hearing that only a minimal number of people had survived this type of cancer was terrifying. I could not look at him; I just kept gazing down at Cassie sleeping peacefully in my arms, contemplating how we could hide our fear and disbelief from the girls. The stillness of the silence was oppressive, and I fought nausea as my brain resonated with questions. How could this be happening? What would become of our family if Greg did not survive? Where would I find the strength to manage this and Rebecca's overwhelming needs? Was this going to be the catalyst to shatter my already fragile mental state?

I have no memory, even after all this time, of walking out of that exam room and back to the girls. The first thing I recall is asking them if they were ready to find some lunch, then, out of habit, asking Stephanie if Rebecca had behaved. I wasn't really concerned about the answer – in that moment the only thing that mattered was not revealing to our young children that life had just kicked the shit out of us in that room. The drive home was quiet, and I could only speculate at what Greg was thinking or feeling because he had shut down the instant the doctor told us the news. He had retreated deep within himself and could not look at the girls or me. Although this situation had petrified me as well, I thought it was necessary to discuss it when we were alone again.

When we got home, I sent the girls out to play as Greg sat in silence, staring into space. Shortly after that, my sister Julie came to pick up Cassie and naturally asked what we found out at the appointment. Greg came to life and adamantly shook his head "no" behind Julie's back, so I said he was referred to a surgeon and nothing more. After she left, Greg was adamant that we keep the cancer from everyone, which I strongly disagreed with. After what turned into a very heated discussion, I grabbed my car keys and told him to watch the girls because I needed to go for a drive. As I rode around, I tried, unsuccessfully, to get a handle on my emotions and to see things from Greg's side. His mandate of hiding the diagnosis from his mom, brother, two sisters, and my family was not acceptable because I felt they had a right to know. Not just that, but we were going to need help with the girls once we saw the surgeon. Before I realized it, I was pulling into the parking lot of the golf course.

I knew Dena was working in the bar that day, and as she was my best friend and constant sidekick, it only made sense that I would seek her out. The golfers were still out on the course, so the bar was empty when I walked in the door. Dena looked up at me, the damn broke, and though it was against Greg's wishes I told her what the doctor had said. She listened as I purged my emotions, then provided the comfort I desperately needed. Dena supported my belief that our families should be told so that they could help us through this ordeal. Promising to keep my secret, she poured me a glass of liquid courage that I sipped until it was time to head home.

Greg is a very private man, and until that day I had always respected his wishes; this time, however, was entirely different. We could not handle this journey without the support of our family and friends, and it was going to be one hell of a battle getting him to accept that reality. Driving home, I was dreading having that conversation because I knew it was going to be an ugly one. Greg and I are both strong, stubborn personalities and neither would back down without a fight.

When I pulled into the drive, the girls were still playing in the backyard, and I told them I was headed in to make dinner. As I did so, I worked through different scenarios, trying to figure out how best to approach Greg.

Conversation during dinner was virtually non-existent, and I wondered whether the girls would think something was wrong. They seemed fine, though, and once we finished, they went back outside to play. I started clearing the dishes and was startled when the ringing phone shattered the stillness; it was Mom Joanne calling to see what Greg had found out at his appointment. Covering the mouthpiece, I told him he was going to tell her or I was, then I handed him the phone. He was still adamantly shaking his head when I left the room and went to get the girls to come inside for their bath. When I later returned to the kitchen, Greg handed me the phone. He told me he had downplayed the situation, only telling her that he was being sent to Mayo Clinic because they suspected cancer. Greg expected me to follow his lead and stood there as I reiterated what he had said and promised to let her know as soon as we had an appointment. It was extremely uncomfortable for me to be deceptive to Mom Joanne but I figured she already knew it was serious if he was being referred to the Mayo Clinic.

I waited until I was sure the girls were asleep, then I sat down with Greg to reopen the discussion. He obstinately insisted that only Mom Joanne was to know. As far as he was concerned, it was his business, and the only thing we could agree upon was that it was best to keep it from the girls as long as possible. Even after I shared the many unknowns about our situation that was robbing me of my piece of mind, it made no impact on his need for secrecy. Who would watch the girls while we were in another state? Where was I going to stay during his operation? What would his recovery entail? Greg seemed unable to accept my need to have emotional and spiritual support to deal with this potentially fatal cancer. Although Greg believes in God, he is not devoted to his Baptist faith or thinks, as I do, being Catholic, that there is power in prayer. As far as I was concerned, we needed all the prayers we could get.

Regardless of my feelings or input, he refused to compromise as we waited for the appointment in Rochester. The waiting was agonizing, and as challenging as it was, I had to agree to wait until Greg choose to tell the family, so long as they were told. He had put up this massive wall and my attempts to get him to open up and share his concerns or fears about having cancer failed.

The silence was damaging, and our once resilient relationship began to show cracks. We moved through each day and took care of our daughters but we were becoming invisible to one another. It was emotionally devastating for me as the fear we lived with wrapped itself tightly around the two of us. We became breathing zombies who sat silently focusing on that big box television so we did not have to interact. Even all the trials and tribulations we'd had with Rebecca never made us incapable of conversing with one another. The girls noticed our abnormal behavior and played outside more, and even though I was aware of the effect it had on them, I was at a loss as to how to fix it.

During those dark days I found myself wishing we'd find our way back to the way we were as newlyweds. Even through our rose-colored lenses, we had learned to work through intense moments by resourcefully adjusting to one another's quirks. We had survived that first disagreement when the boxing gloves of politeness came off and a tremendous fight ensued. Days went by with us scarcely speaking to one another as we held on to our "badges of honor" that were really all about pride and stupidity. Of course, that intensified the situation and created petty grievances. We realized that in order to repair our relationship, we first had to melt the icy silence. That awareness gave us the insight that our anger stemmed from the inability to read each other's minds. Once we cooled our tempers, we were able to stop inflicting pain on each other and instead wait until we could calmly and candidly discuss our emotions.

Looking back, I think the essential wisdom we gained was that our personal imperfections were merely human qualities and not opportunities to criticize. The difference between then and now was that we were facing a crisis that could not be fixed by an apology or a kiss. In the throes of this potentially life-ending crisis, we had lost our ability to be vulnerable and share our feelings. We had lost our sense of being partners and working together; we let the fear paralyze us into slipping farther away from one other. Thankfully, in time we not only resolved the problem but strategized about how to deal with these situations in the future.

It took almost two weeks before the Mayo Clinic contacted us for an appointment. They advised us that it would be one day of testing, and we would receive the results the following day. That meant we would need to spend the night in Rochester. Since my parents had moved to California, I asked my sister Cindy and her husband Mike to take care of the girls. It took some determined arm-twisting, but Greg finally permitted me to share our secret with them. Having an appointment seemed to get him to reengage with life again, and I think it was because the limbo of waiting was over. We would soon have the answers to our many questions and hopefully, get the surgery scheduled.

We had moments of comfortable conversation as Greg drove to Minnesota, and I latched on to that as an encouraging sign for our relationship. It was relatively easy to locate the Mayo Clinic, considering it was a vast complex compared to our small-town medical center. With the various floors and multiple elevators, it was like entering a completely different dimension. Given the massive amount of people there we could see why they had told us it would be an entire day of testing. When Greg finally got through the check-in procedure, we took a seat in the large waiting room while they compiled his paperwork necessary for each department. There were substantial sized waiting rooms for the laboratory and x-ray departments, and they called out for six people at a time. It reminded me of the herding of animals the way they bunched up the patients into groups before taking them back for the test. Yes, the small townsfolk was definitely coming out in me as I stared awestruck at this well-oiled machine of a medical facility.

I utilized the waiting time to pray, thanking God that Greg's first doctor was assertive enough to get him into this clinic. We had entered the building in the morning, and when Greg was finished it was late afternoon, and being famished we went searching for an inexpensive place to eat. This was not easy, for though the food choices in the area were abundant they had prices to match the epic reputation of the impressive Mayo Clinic. After we finished eating, our next stop was to find an economical motel. Greg headed away from the complex and eventually located one out by the interstate. It was affordable; unfortunately, it was also in desperate need of repairs, updating, and fumigation.

Greg was satisfied that since it was only for one night, it would be sufficient, but I was not as convinced. Our banter seemed less strained as long as we chatted about other things besides why we were sitting in that dreary motel. When it came time to turn off the lights, I expressed my concern, saying that more than likely there would be critters coming out once we did. Greg laughed at me as he went over to lock the door and stopped laughing when he discovered that the lock was broken. Nothing to worry about, he assured me as he dropped our overnight bag in front of the door to give us a warning if someone tried to enter. He then quickly dropped off to sleep, while I, fully dressed and sitting upright, kept my eyes glued to the door as scenes from Hitchcock movies flashed through my mind. From time to time, I would be snapped awake by the pain in my neck as my head dropped to my chest. It was, needless to say, a very long night for me.

Morning finally arrived, and I could not get out of that place fast enough; I also prayed we had not taken any "hitchhikers" with us in our hasty exit. Since we had ample time before our next appointment at Mayo, we went in search of breakfast to recharge our bodies. Grabbing muffins and coffee from a little shop, we enjoyed the sunshine and quiet morning as we looked at storefronts. Our slow and steady steps fell into a rhythm as we walked silently side by side with our thoughts about the results that awaited our return. Off in the distance, we spotted a bench and the perfect spot to finish our coffee and people watch. The birds serenaded us as the bees buzzed the flowers, and the silence that fell between us was again comfortable. We were not eager to relinquish the gift that nature was providing when it was time to start our walk over to the glass doors of the Mayo Clinic.

When we met with the doctor, he patiently explained that the tests performed the day before had confirmed the first doctor's diagnosis of cancer. He also told us that the tumor, which was attached to the back of Greg's knee, had been there for quite some time. The shock came when he told us that it was imperative that surgery be performed the next day. He was very clear that the tests only told him part of the story and it wasn't until he made the incision that he would know exactly what the procedure would entail or what the outcome would be. Most terrifying was the revelation that if the tumor were to get a puncture it would prove fatal for Greg.

The surgeon's first objective was to discover how the tumor was attached to his knee. If it were not encased to the knee, then he would need to extract it very carefully. If the tumor was encased around the knee, the extraction would entail a partial femur and knee rebuild. Then the doctor took a deep breath, looked directly at Greg, and stated the worst-case scenario: if it was unsafe to remove the tumor he would have no other choice but to amputate the leg above the knee. At that point it would be his only chance of saving Greg's life.

CHAPTER SEVEN

The Fork in the Road

"We must let go of the life we have planned to accept the one that is waiting for us."

Joseph Campbell

It was a lot to digest, and although the doctor had given us a clearer understanding of the surgery, it still left us with an unknown outcome. Would Greg survive? As we left the exam room in an emotional fog, we headed down the hallway to the small door-less phone cubicles. Greg talked softly to Mom Joanne as he told her about his impending surgery, and since she was coming, spared her the details until she arrived. Mom Joanne had asked him to get her a motel room next to ours, and since there was no way we were going to return to that grimy, unsecured, and possibly flea-infested hovel, we went in search of better lodgings that could accommodate us all. After Mom Joanne arrived, we headed to dinner; there, she admitted that she had called Greg's siblings. He was still not comfortable with them knowing his condition but at this point there was nothing he could do about it.

Our meal was a subdued affair with our thoughts focused on the surgery, and we retired to our rooms early, hoping Greg could get a good night's sleep. Just as I was getting ready to head into the bathroom, the phone rang, and it was Greg's younger brother Mark. They chatted for a minute before Greg handed me the phone saying Mark wanted to talk to me. I figured he would be upset, and sure enough, he chastised me for not calling him. Greg's need for privacy had put me right where I knew it would, with family and friends automatically holding me accountable for them being kept in the dark about his cancer. Before our conversation ended, he had my word of honor that from that point forward, he would be updated immediately with all the facts.

There was no way to change how things happened, and loving Mark as I did, I did not take it personally. I handed the phone back to Greg and went into the bathroom. With my poker face of optimism in place, I came out and got into bed and prayed for a dreamless sleep. I woke up refreshed and thankful for the gift since I had lost so much sleep from our night at Motel Sketchy. Greg was up and dressed and snipped at me to get moving, so our day started on a surly note. We met up with Mom Joanne and headed over to the hospital for Greg to be prepped for surgery. He was settled in bed when the nurse informed us that his operation had been moved to later in the afternoon, which understandably worsened his mood. As the lunch hour rolled around, Greg insisted we leave and find something to eat since he could not. We stopped by the nurse's station to inquire about the time for his surgery and discovered it had been pushed back again.

Due to the second delay in Greg's surgery, it was close to midnight before we learned the outcome. The surgeon told us that he had been successful at removing the tumor without it rupturing. Unfortunately, to accomplish that feat, he'd had to do an extensive leg repair and a knee replacement, but I could only be grateful that he had not had to remove the leg altogether.

It was not an easy recovery. Greg was in tremendous pain and after the first few days, quite agitated. Being in the room with him was a lot like trying to maneuver around hidden landmines. The staff did their best to make the pain tolerable, but his surgery had been so substantial that he was already on the highest dose of pain med. He also had multiple drain tubes and required constant care. Once the tubes were removed, he would be moved to another ward to continue his recovery.

Upon hearing this news, it put us all into an emotional tailspin, as we had assumed we would be going home together. My emotional duress was much like being trapped inside a snow globe scurrying around trying to grab the falling flakes to keep them from burying me alive. Mom Joanne and Cindy both needed to return to work, so that necessitated my return home. My Catholic guilt kicked in and made me feel sick about deserting Greg, but there was no other choice. The girls were delighted to see me, and Cindy did not appear too exhausted from caring for our energized Rebecca. There was some measure of comfort having a routine to keep me busy, and I tried to stay upbeat so the girls would not realize how dangerous this surgery had been for their dad. There were never enough hours in the day as I tried to keep up with the girls and my daycare and I was so appreciative that at least I was able to take time off from my night job.

The challenges didn't end when Greg was released from the hospital. His illness, and the resulting loss of his income, had promoted me to breadwinner and head of the family. As for the girls, they were just relieved to have him home. While I was relieved as well, his return also added to my already overloaded plate. I had his care, the girls, my daycare and my night job, which we badly needed to pay the bills. Though my income was far less than Greg's, it kept the creditors at bay, which was our primary concern. To say the stress took a toll on my charming personality is being polite. While chatting on the phone with Mom, she strongly suggested that before school started we should come to California for a visit.

As the saying goes, once a parent always a parent. Mom understood I needed a reprieve from the abundant load I shouldered, and she and Dad were more than willing to take some of that weight from me. We even found time for fun. Dad insisted we spend a day at Disney Land and arranged a wheelchair for Greg because his cast went from the top his thigh down to his toes. Of course, Greg, who hates attention of any kind, disliked this idea, but the rest of us appreciated being advanced to the head of the lines. It sure made the theme park more enjoyable in the hot sun and gave Rebecca an advantage by riding on her dad's lap when she got tired. The chair handles were also useful for the big dangling purse with Rebecca's food items. She was incredible about staying true to her diet without any grumbling.

Rebecca saw the Magic Carpet ride and started nagging for me to take her up the steep flight of stairs for what amounted to a ride down on a scratchy burlap bag. When she was undeterred by my firm no, her Papa told her she was big enough to go by herself and did not need me. He didn't have to say it twice. Rebecca ran to grab a carpet and climbed the stairs, while I turned to Dad and asked why the hell he'd told her that because now I would have to get her when she chickened out.

We watched as she spread out the burlap, tucked in her feet as instructed, and then froze. The employee tried to get her to slide down, but she refused to budge, so he looked down at us for help. I gave dad my *told you so* face, and he told me to stay put because he was going to bring her down. Ignoring my concern for his bad back, Dad strolled off, climbed the stairs, and sat down behind Rebecca as he put his arms around her. He whispered something in her ear and then pushed them off, and they could have caught bugs in their teeth with the mammoth smiles on their faces!

I roared with laughter as they slid to a stop where I stood, and the pure moment of joy in watching my daddy and little girl having such tremendous fun uplifted my heart and spirit. My little manic jumped up with excitement, and Dad handed her the rug to take back, then came over to me and gave me a tight squeeze.

As he kissed my cheek, he said, "My sore ass from that damn ride was well worth it, Butch, to see you laugh like that."

Though my parents had named me after Dad's only sister, he had given me the nickname Butch because I had been born bald and slow to grow hair. I can never recall Dad calling me anything but Butch. It still amazes me that even after all this time, that memory of the carpet ride can always make me smile and feel my daddy's love.

On the way out of Disney Land, the girls got helium balloons, and the next day Greg asked Dad if he had ever inhaled helium. When he said he had never heard of such a thing, Stephanie quickly offered up her balloon. Greg inhaled the gas and talked to Dad with his Mickey Mouse voice. Dad laughed so darn hard that tears leaked out of his eyes, and it was hilarious watching him get that much amusement from this discovery. He could barely contain his excitement at having his turn, and those two had tremendous fun deflating the girl's balloons. We laughed so much that our sides hurt from all that joy. We could never express the depth of our love or appreciation to my parents for the magnitude of healing they gave our family during that visit.

The carefree spirit of summer was coming to an end, and we faced the drudgery of shopping for clothes and supplies in preparation for another schoolyear. As usual, the girls enjoyed the thrill of the hunt for new clothes, shoes, school bags, and all the trappings that shrunk our already depleted checkbook. My focus was on wearing out my rosary beads, this time praying for a good teacher for Rebecca. Other than that week with the folks, my emotional stability was again unpredictable, and I woke up some mornings with an awful feeling of dread. I struggled to make it through those days, waiting for the moment I could fall into bed, emotionally exhausted. At least my prayers seemed to be answered when we learned Rebecca's second-grade teacher was Delpha, a neighbor to Mom Joanne. According to the parent rumor mill, she was an excellent teacher, and there was a glimmer of hope on the horizon.

Delpha was approachable and open to my request to be part of her team and help Rebecca adapt to the second grade. The year started with promise, only for my optimism to be shattered with the notification that her academic struggles were mirroring those of first grade. Rebecca was having difficulty following directions, completing the work, and struggling enough that Delpha felt the AEA should implement an evaluation.

Added to this was the news that a problem had developed in the healing of Greg's leg and he needed to return to Minnesota for a second surgery. The urge to hit the booze was never stronger than at that moment, even knowing from experience that it would change nothing and only create more shit for me to deal with. It took everything I had not to give in to that urge and thank goodness I did not because I might have missed a sign that something was up with Stephanie.

When we explained that her dad needed surgery again, our usually outgoing and happy daughter started to withdraw. Knowing how intuitive she was, I attempted to get her to share with me, but all she would do was parrot that she was fine. Obviously, this was not the case so I asked my sister Pat, a nurse in psychiatry, to chat with her. Pat later confirmed my suspicion that Stephanie had surmised that Greg's medical needs were far more severe than we let on; in fact she was terrified that he was dying. I sat her down and reassured her that Greg was not dying, and that the additional surgery was so the doctor could make his leg stronger. Though that news seemed to comfort her, I was still concerned. At this point, I had all the balls in the air and lacked the skills to keep them there.

This time around, my brother Jim and his girlfriend Donna stayed at the house with the girls so their school schedule wouldn't be interrupted. Greg and I headed to Minnesota for the surgery, and since there was a complication brewing at school with Rebecca, I would stay only until he was stable then return home. At the end of the week, I would pick up the girls from school and drive to Minnesota to see Greg. Thankfully, the hospital provided a TV and VCR so I brought along movies for our entertainment.

It was while Rebecca was on the bed cuddling with Greg that I noticed her eyes roll up behind her eyelids and then down again. My first thought was that it was some type of nervous tick from all the turmoil and stress created by Greg's surgeries. It had not been easy for the girls being left in the care of different family members for days, and now they were enduring long car rides to see their dad.

My common sense tried to convince me there was nothing to worry about and stop fretting because I already had enough on my plate. When it happened several more times, my instinct kicked in, relentless in its warnings of upcoming turmoil, just as it had done since I was about the age of nine.

Once we got Greg home and settled, I contacted our doctor about the eye rolling, and he referred us to a neurologist. An EEG was performed, and Rebecca was suffering from petit mal seizures and needed to be placed on medication. Within a few days of taking the medicine, Rebecca displayed an increase in hyperactivity and complained of severe headaches. I called the neurologist with my belief that the red dye in the medication was causing these problems, but he disregarded my theory, saying that the medication Rebecca was taking was also used to manage migraine headaches.

Here again, I was at odds with a physician, but Rebecca had been free of chemicals for over two years and I was not going to undo all we had accomplished. When I refused to back down he did prescribe a medication without dyes but failed to instruct me to decrease the doses of the first medication, rather than abruptly stopping it. This lack of information caused Rebecca to experience her first grand mal seizure, which prompted a referral to a neurologist at Iowa Medical Center in Des Moines. The new neurologist believed that the eye rolling was a sign of a tic rather than a sign of a seizure disorder, and being mindful of my request, prescribed medication without artificial dyes. The new drug was in capsules that I pulled apart to dispense the white crystals onto a spoon of ice cream, and within three days the headaches stopped, the hyperactivity decreased, and Rebecca was once again calm.

Indeed, life seemed hellbent on not giving me an inch. One day, the dreaded phone rang, and this time, it was a social worker from AEA calling to request an in-home visit. They sent Mike, a kind young man who during the conversation referred to his evaluation of Rebecca while at school. To say we were shocked was an understatement. Given our previous history with the AEA, I was also suspicious. My initial mistrust of the AEA had occurred when I discovered we needed their permission to have Rebecca attend kindergarten in the public-school system.

Now an evaluation had taken place without our knowledge, which was against protocol. I aired my displeasure to Mike, and though he said he was unaware that we had not been notified, I remained distrustful. After he left, I vented to Greg, who said he felt we should give them the benefit of the doubt. Part of me wondered if his detached attitude was just Greg being Greg (and avoiding conflict at all costs), or because he was busy preparing for a trip west to see his brother Mark.

Mark was building a house in Washington state, and now that Greg was back on his feet he had sent him tickets to fly out there and help with the plumbing. A few days after Greg left, a letter arrived from the AEA, notifying us of a conference scheduled at Butler School. That evening I called Greg and shared with him about the meeting and my reluctance to attend without him. He listened to my misgivings and then assured me that my "bad vibes" were probably due to exhaustion. This answer gave me absolutely no comfort because Greg was never comfortable hearing about my premonitions and thought them weird.

He went on to say, in his matter of fact tone, that my emotions were most likely the result of dealing with issues revolving around Rebecca and his surgeries. I just didn't realize how much everything had affected me. His calm logical words felt like a slap across the face. How the hell could he think I was unaware of the effect those stressors had been to my mental and physical health? Just as I was about to blast him with an angry rebuttal, he told me how much he respected and admired me for handling all that responsibility. Hearing my man of few words say those things deflated my indignation; it also saddened me to listen to him confesses how tough and painful it had been to watch me carry all that weight alone. Our conversation ended with him trying to convince me that everything would be fine, but my instincts still warned that I was walking into an ambush.

I walked into the principal's office that day with a mask of friendless on my face and ominous vibrations running throughout my body. Aside from myself and the principal, Rebecca's teacher, Mike, and another representative from the AEA were in attendance. Once the introductions were made, the AEA representative took the lead and enlightened me regarding the most recent evaluation done on Rebecca. The issues, as they saw them, involved her seizures, the hyperactivity, difficulty with visual perception; it was these conditions that were interfering with her academic progress. Also, her adaptive behavior in and out of school was below average, and therefore, the AEA would be changing her primary disability of Communicative Learning Disabled to Mentally Disabled.

This bewildered me, since none of the multiple physicians treating Rebecca ever stated she exhibited signs of a mental disability. When I told them that I objected to the new diagnosis and asked how these symptoms could now be so severe when she had achieved academic success in kindergarten and acquired the ability to read, my questions were ignored and a parental consent form was slid across the desk. Then they informed me that once I signed, thereby agreeing to the label Mentally Disabled, Rebecca would be removed from Butler and placed across town in a different school. It was 1991, and their solution for children who like Rebecca did not function well in a regular classroom was to remove and seclude them. As much as they tried to present it as an improved solution for Rebecca, everything in me was telling me otherwise.

With extreme determination and fighting back tears, I stated that I disagreed with both the diagnosis and the placement and refused to sign. I then stood up and walked out. My whole body was shaking, and I barely made it to the outside before my vision blurred and I tasted the salt from tears streaming down my face. Walking as fast as I could without appearing to run, I headed to the car and was almost there when I heard someone was calling my name. Quickly wiping my face, I turned around to find Mike standing there. He asked me to wait so he could talk to me, and if it had been anyone else but him, I would not have stopped.

Mike expressed how deeply sorry he was for my pain, then stated it was imperative that I understood the techniques and tests that they used in evaluations. These were merely tools to assist them in determining a diagnosis and that none of them had all the answers. The one thing Mike was confident about after spending time with Rebecca and me was that she would succeed in life because she had my fighting spirit. He told me to keep kicking down doors on her behalf, and I embraced his words of encouragement. Mike's deep conviction in my strength and ability was my greatest motivation not to quit.

Once I had myself composed, I called Greg to give him the details of the meeting and that I had been spot-on about it being an ambush. As usual, I vented and told him I was adamant that unless a specialist validated the AEA finding of Mental Disability, I would not sign that consent form. Knowing he was fighting a losing battle, he suggested I contact our physician. The doctor in turn referred us to the University Hospital in Iowa City, which had a Pediatric Department of Developmental Disabilities. When Greg returned from Washington, he seemed aloof, and I attributed it to being tired. The next night in bed, he pulled me close, and naturally, I presumed it was snuggling time. Instead, he blindsided me by asking if I would consider moving to Washington.

My heart began to race as I fought the urge to run from the dark bedroom. When I remained mute, Greg softly asked what I was thinking and, still stunned by his request, all I could utter was that I needed time. I then rolled over and placed my back to him like a wall of defense. The next sound I heard was his wavering voice, saying he knew it was asking a lot of me, but he needed me to agree so that he could try to rebuild his life. The leg surgery had robbed him of his trade as a plumber and unfortunately our hometown did not offer much in the way of management positions for his expertise. He had secured a job after the surgery, but they let him go because the limited stability of his leg was a liability. It had been a severe blow to his self-esteem, and though I knew his request to move was not unreasonable it nevertheless led to a full-fledged panic.

Except for my parents and one sister, all my siblings, extended family members, and friends would have to be left behind. Relinquishing my entire support system was petrifying. Although Greg had provided exceptional financial care of our family, he had never been very demonstrative when it came to his emotions. I had thought once we were married he would become more comfortable showing affection, but he never could allow himself to be that vulnerable. Being an affectionate person, I had grown to depend on family and friends to provide me with that security. Greg had family waiting in Washington, and as deeply as I loved Mark, it felt like I was the only one being asked to give up so much for this opportunity. Suddenly, I found myself in a tug of war between the lifeline of people I relied on and the love of my life who was dying inside day by day. It was an excruciating choice, and I deeply identified with the statement "A heart is breaking into pieces" because mine came damn close.

As I was wrestling with my conflicting emotions, I learned that the plan for our move was much more developed than Greg had originally revealed. In fact, he, Mark and Yolanda had apparently worked out several logistics during his visit. The house would be ready for Mark, Yolanda, their three-year-old daughter Jaci, and four-month-old son Ben to move into by the time we arrived. We would live on their property in the fifth-wheel trailer while Greg worked with Job Source to locate a job. In exchange for us living there, I would take care of Jaci and Ben, just as I provided childcare for my siblings now. To say that my Irish was a wee bit ticked off was an understatement! The feelings of betrayal that Greg would discuss a significant decision in our lives without my knowledge, input, or even my presence, were immense. In the end, though, "for better or worse" won out and we loaded up the U-Haul and my car and headed west to start our lives all over again.

Greg also felt that we should sign the new diagnosis to appease the AEA and Butler. He believed it would not hurt Rebecca to be placed temporarily in the Mentally Disabled classroom, but I strongly disagreed. My conviction was that endorsing the placement, without a medical confirmation of a mental disability, was unfair to Rebecca and would label her for life. I stood firm on my principles and refused to sign, so Greg did and she spent several weeks in that school before we moved. On December 5, 1991, family and friends came to help load us up and say goodbye. It was a weepy drive for us girls as we followed Greg and drove away from all we had ever known.

We hit a whiteout in Montana that necessitated us finding a motel for the night, so we didn't arrive until nearly midnight the following night. The next morning my stomach rolled over as I saw our new digs for the first time. The trailer was a far cry from our two-story house back in Iowa and I, being claustrophobic, had no idea how I would deal with it. Clearly, it would be a tremendous adjustment and require an abundance of patience. The pullout couch became our new bed, and there was just enough room on the floor of the overhang area for the girl's mattresses. We shared one closet, and several cubbies for our minimal clothing and the small TV sat on the kitchen table with only room for two chairs. The rest of our belongings were stored in Mark's basement until the day we once again had a house.

There was limited space in the kitchen with only room for essential kitchenware, and next to the kitchen was the bathroom "closet." And a closet it was, with just enough room for a small shallow tub and shower combo, a sink, and a small commode. The water heater was tiny, so we had to take extremely quick showers or boil enough water for a bath. After the second round of that bullshit I began using the tub at the big house. As if adapting to this new living arrangement were not challenging enough, Greg and Stephanie both developed bronchitis, which necessitated us finding a doctor immediately. It was a miracle that Rebecca and I dodged those nasty germs while living in such close quarters. Once Stephanie was healthy again, she was enrolled in the sixth grade at Stanwood Middle School and Rebecca into second grade at Twin City Elementary.

The specialized education staff at Twin City School disagreed with the Mental Disability diagnosis by the AEA and placed Rebecca in a regular second-grade classroom with assistance from the Special Education Department. Linda was an excellent teacher with her expertise and dedication being instrumental in helping Rebecca excel; it was an encouraging development and the first favorable thing about moving. We had a bit of an adjustment to the quaint little town that had yet to evolve to the point of installing a stoplight (there was only a flashing yellow light overhead by the fire station). It was as if we had crossed more than a time zone when we left behind our industrial hometown and entered this rural place that seemed to have changed little in the past God knows how many years.

The main street was maybe two blocks in length with a minimal number of storefronts and limited selections of merchandise. There was a police station, a small clothing store, drug store, grocery store, and hardware store. Down from Main Street was a post office, small medical center, library, two gas stations, the middle school, and one of the elementary schools. Up the hill from downtown were the high school, another elementary school, a senior living center, and a small malt shop. The town was closed each night by 10:00 p.m. and no one worked on Sundays so folks could worship, which was nice but a culture shock for the four of us.

We were just beginning to embrace our new life when two weeks later the other shoe dropped. My mom suffered a severe stroke that was going to require surgery, and the prognosis was not very encouraging. The doctor told Dad it was unlikely she would survive the surgery so my siblings were headed to California. Suddenly, my heart was being ripped apart all over again. How could I leave the girls so soon after uprooting them and with Christmas a week away? On the other hand, the thought of losing my mom, and that I might not be there, was killing me. Knowing that, Greg insisted I fly to California. He felt confident that he could care for the girls, especially since Yolanda had offered to help. It seemed like too much to ask since we were only starting to get to know one another, but in the end I knew I had to go.

I flew to California in time to see mom before surgery, and she came through retaining her ability to speak, though it was apparent she had limitations. There were issues with her short-term memory and weakness in her limbs; it would also take some time before her speech returned to normal. Yet I never doubted her ability to heal because she was a fighter who never embraced quitting.

Mom would sometimes get irritated with what she called my "stubborn spirit," to which I would counter that I had gotten it from her genes and therefore was not responsible for it. She was an inspiration as she diligently worked to regain her strength and taught herself to read again. It was difficult for her to accept that she could no longer work or drive, and Dad did his best to take on more of the responsibilities. Within a few years, they would move back home to Iowa, where Dad had the support of my siblings.

When I returned from California the girls were excited to fill me in about Christmas, and how their dad had cut a large evergreen limb for their Christmas tree. Greg put it in a bucket of sand on the table, and the girls made decorations the old-fashioned way as he played Santa, apparently with assistance. Yolanda had invited them to join her side of the family for Christmas, and that helped dissipate some of my guilt at not being there. We rang in the New Year and settled into a routine of the girls getting ready to meet the school bus, Greg heading off to Job Source, and me walking up to the "big house" to take care of Jaci and Ben. Life seemed to be back on solid ground and showing the promise of happiness, which was a blessing after we had gone through so much upheaval in the last year.

Six months later, school ended, and it was a beautiful six months of no phone calls and having an extraordinary teacher. Linda and her husband hosted the year-end class party, parents included, at their cabin on the water, which was such a generous gift. The kids had a blast fishing, taking turns going out on the boat, and it was just an overall pleasant experience with which to end the schoolyear. Having a chance to get to know other parents helped us blend more comfortably into our new community. Greg was working at a glass factory, and after seven months, we moved out of the trailer into an old modular home that we had purchased. Two steps forward and one step back, though because the move placed us in a different school district, just as Rebecca was getting ready to begin third grade.

Our luck held steady, and Rebecca's third-grade teacher, also named Lisa, had the same caliber of skill in assisting Rebecca to succeed academically. During spring break, I took the girls to see my folks in

California, and while on an amusement ride, Rebecca was sideswiped. She complained of hip pain, so I took her to the doctor and discovered she had a congenital disability of her hips that required surgery to insert screws in both. Rebecca was a resilient warrior like her dad and grandma and recovered quickly with slight limitations in the rotation of her hips. She looked forward to going back to school since she was catching up and just about within the normal range of grade expectations. On her progress report, Linda wrote, "Rebecca's cheerfulness and thoughtfulness brighten the day. She always has a kind word for someone and is ready to help someone in need. Because of Rebecca, the other students have learned to overcome some of their aches and pains, and everyone in the room is proud of her. It has been a good year for Rebecca, I have enjoyed her projects and comments, and she certainly is a caring and dependable young lady. It has been my pleasure to have her in my class." From that uplifting note, we both looked forward to fourth grade with high expectations.

The following schoolyear got off to a hopeful start, but things seemed to get progressively harder for her. She was struggling, and it was concluded the best thing was to place her in the Resource Room for reading and math. Rebecca never made enough progress to return fulltime to the regular classroom. With two teachers it was a challenge for me to keep up with the communication, but Rebecca appeared happy and content. My request for open contact with the teachers was never about control; it was an alert system for academic or behavioral problems with Rebecca. It was problematic to give her consequences for bad choices when I heard about them days or weeks later. Thank goodness the only ongoing behavioral issue was her not staying on task. My role at this point was to give support with homework and prepare her for tests. Rebecca did her best to please everyone, which was remarkable, considering she was coping with the expectations of multiple adults at one time!

With fifth grade looming on the horizon, I finally accepted that there was no point in stressing about what obstacles or struggles

Rebecca would encounter. I would have to adapt to a different teacher and different learning and communication challenges and accept that things might be a continuation of what we had already been through. My focus was on making sure that she did not fall behind and I learned to embrace the idea that her progress in the next grade would be successful regardless of how much time she spent in Special Education. Fifth grade started the same as fourth grade, with her having consistent struggles within the regular classroom and therefore placed for the same number of hours in Special Education. As I learned to ride each wave as it came, I realized that my mindset definitely made a difference in how smoothly the year went.

By sixth grade, I was determined to ensure a better transition and outcome at the middle school. I contacted the principal and requested a meeting with him and all of Rebecca's teachers so that I could convey my desire to work side by side with them as they tended to Rebecca's academic and social needs. Present at the meeting were the Vice Principle, the Life Skills teacher, the Spelling teacher, the Social Studies teacher, and the Health teacher. They were appreciative of my commitment and receptive to developing a team effort to help Rebecca reach her full potential. When I left that meeting, I was extremely confident that these individuals were just as determined as I to create a learning plan for success.

Unlike the past two years, Rebecca would be placed in Life Skills, which was the Special Education Department, for Math and Reading and regular classes with a teacher's aide for Spelling, Health, and Social Studies. Since the bus ride home from school was relatively long, Rebecca had a chance to unwind and be ready to sit down at the table with her snack and do homework. The aide sent information to help me prepare Rebecca for any upcoming tests, and I helped with homework if it was necessary. All her tests were given orally since she learned best that way, and using this system was working exceptionally well. Then one day I walked out the mailbox, found a letter from the school, and instantly thought, "Oh crap!" Though as far as I knew everything was fine at school, it was never good news to get correspondence in the mail. I let it sit on the counter for a while because I was too scared to open it.

My curiosity finally prevailed, and I ripped it open quickly, like ripping off a bandage, to read what was inside. Unfolding the single sheet of paper, I read, "Your student has demonstrated academic excellence with an honor roll grade point of 3.6 or above. This places them in the Highest Honor Club, and we would like to congratulate your student and proudly invite them to attend a celebration party in their honor."

Holy shit! Our perseverance enabled Rebecca to make the honor roll! I yelled for Rebecca, who came out of her room with a slightly perplexed look on her face. I read the letter to her, and we jumped around the kitchen as if we had won the lottery. It was a surreal moment, and we were still in high spirits two hours later when Greg got home. That personal achievement boosted Rebecca's self-esteem and gave her the self-confidence to believe she was capable of learning. She had achieved this tremendous success from her diligence at learning the material, and the unwavering support of her teachers, aides, and myself. For the first time since third grade, there was validation that a team effort positively made a difference!

The most incredible outcome of her making the honor roll was in her realizing that she was equal to the other students. Although she learned the information differently than her classmates, she had accomplished what many students had not. Something deep inside of her seemed to awaken as she realized she was just as worthy as her peers of academic excellence. Rebecca seemed to bloom from that point, and it made my heart sing. If there were any lingering regrets about leaving Iowa, they no longer existed. Both of us had flourished tremendously on this journey, and I doubt we could have reached this pinnacle in life if we had not moved. The saying, "What does not kill you makes you stronger," was never more apparent than watching her attain such joy academically.

What would have happened to her if we had stayed in Iowa? Would my fight for her have failed? I cannot predict what I do not know, but there is little doubt that everything we went through was for this celebration. What I have concluded is that our family transformed and prospered significantly from the intense squalls that blew into our lives and pushed us onward, through the storm, to the immense possibilities upon the shores of Washington. If not for those life-changing circumstances, we may have never felt compelled to take a leap of faith that has brought us more joy than pain. Even with the trials and tribulations, I cannot imagine our family living anywhere else and have faith that our beautiful state of Washington still has an abundance of possibilities yet to be discovered.

CHAPTER EIGHT

Maneuvering the School Years

"Pain nourishes courage. You can't be brave if you've only had wonderful things happen to you."

Mary Tyler Moore

Seventh grade began with a different teacher in the Life Skills Classroom, which meant starting all over again to build a respectful and productive partnership. Transitioning into the next grade level is so much easier with the same people in place. Rebecca always did better academically when she returned to the teachers and aides from the year before, and the reliable strategies already implemented. That said, I found Kim, the new teacher, an asset to the Special Education program. She was a strong advocate for her students who went into other classrooms and adamant that class time was primary and field trips were secondary. I certainly appreciated her stand on limited field trips because we were sending Rebecca to school for a curriculum in academics and not for various outings off campus.

The year went smoothly, and to our joy and relief Rebecca continued to make progress. So when toward the end of the schoolyear Kim confided in me that she would not be returning, I went into panic mode. Rebecca was doing so well, and I feared Kim's leaving would make a negative impact. She reassured me that there was nothing to worry about and that she would provide a detailed outline of each student's program strategies for the incoming teacher. I genuinely appreciated that, but – though I am now appalled to admit it - I could not muster genuine happiness for her. Call it selfishness, call it desperation - I just wanted continued success for my daughter, and stability was a key ingredient.

That stability would be threatened further when just before eighth grade began we were notified of a restructuring within the Special Education Department. Rebecca was being moved to the newly built Middle School. At the open house, Greg and I made a point of introducing ourselves to Chad, the new teacher, and expressed our desire to set up a meeting and discuss strategies for Rebecca's academic program. He asked us to give him about two weeks since he was new to this position, and once he had things set up he would call.

After we left school, I confided to Greg that I was apprehensive about Chad's amiable and docile demeanor. People with those personality traits were precisely the ones Rebecca felt compelled to manipulate, and even though many of her behavioral issues had improved with the diet, that specific personality quirk persisted. I envisioned her playing similar mind games with Chad as she had with Carl, the psychologist from AEA. Chad seemed a lot like Carl, and he too would be oblivious to the fact that Rebecca saw him not as an educator but as an adversary. Greg was also concerned with Chad's delicate disposition and felt that we might be in for a rough year, at least relative to the last one.

It took several weeks, but as promised Chad reached out to me to set up an appointment. I enlightened him to Rebecca's "behavioral survival strategies," which encompassed a stubborn streak and extraordinary skill at manipulation. Since these behaviors had been problematic in the past, it was imperative that there be consistent communication between school and home. Chad merely smiled and declared that he was more than capable of handling her personality; he also implied that he would be open to us having an interaction *if necessary*. He was confident that his aide Christine would work well with Rebecca since she had worked well with other students and teachers. Then he condescendingly told me not to worry one little bit about it! Yep, I left that meeting trying to figure out the best way to avoid or deal with the shitstorm I knew was coming. History was about to repeat itself, and it was going to be like preschool all over again.

Any time a teacher felt the need to impress upon me that they were highly capable, knowledgeable, and equipped to handle students like Rebecca, it never ended well for anyone. They all assumed I was unaware that certain behaviors were typical of all kids, when in truth they did not comprehend that my child did not fit or play even close to the usual mold. Chad started out providing open communication, but then he began to falter. Days would go by before he would notify me of a problem. I tried again to get him to recognize that the delay in contacting me about her inappropriate behavior made it extremely challenging to give Rebecca consequences. How was I supposed to effectively discipline her three or four days after an infraction? Whether he realized it or not, Chad's failure to promptly notify me of problems was allowing Rebecca to continue with her rebellious antics and thwart his authority. It felt as though Chad had given me a lengthy prison sentence without any possibility of parole.

My frustration with Rebecca's battles was reminiscent of my own school days. Like her, though not as severe, I too had difficulty learning, and some of the teachers were impatient and unkind about it. I never provoked them, but only because that would have resulted in some painful discipline at the hands of my mom. It left me with little choice other than to suffer in silence. Back then, teachers were unaware of learning disabilities; children who presented a challenge were considered brain damaged and usually did not attended regular schools. The extremely slow learners were held back to repeat a grade, and apparently, I did not fit into either of those categories. This made school a dreadful struggle for me as I tried to understand and process the information – always barely passing and always advanced to the next grade where I was at a significant disadvantage. This endless attempt to catch up caused me untold stress and caused me to despise school intensely.

As a result of my experiences and challenges, I had a tremendous fear of Rebecca attending high school while struggling to attain the necessary academics. Like me, she battled trying to achieve the knowledge of her current grade level only to move to the next while still being behind. Her mental development was more compromised than mine was, as my primary deficit had concerned my social skills. Rarely was I accepted by my peers, so school was a constant and tormenting endeavor that brought more pain than pleasure. It was solely through the efforts of my family, a few dedicated teachers, and my dear friend Jackie that I was able to graduate high school. College was never on my radar. I lacked the desire and the money, and literally tossed off my cap and gown after graduation and hit the pavement looking for full-time employment.

The communication problem with Chad persisted as Rebecca frequently challenged his authority. Though she did behave well for Christine and the teachers in the regular classroom, I was out of patience. I made an appointment with the school psychologist and requested an evaluation on Rebecca hoping that he might provide helpful strategies to correct the problem. He implemented the assessment and mailed me a copy of his report along with his suggestions. Chad would create a folder for Rebecca with his daily communication to me, which she would be responsible for taking home each day. I was to sign the report and any homework assignments and continue working with Chad to resolve any further problems. The psychologist then informed me that Rebecca had confided she was frustrated with my expectation of her doing her homework right after school and that it was too demanding. What child does not find a parent demanding?

After reading his behavioral report, I did wonder if she had a point and I was being too demanding about homework being done right away. The thought did enter my mind that Rebecca was playing puppeteer again, but since I was uncertain, I decided to let her choose when she wanted to do her homework. Of course, she preferred doing it after dinner, which was concerning for me because her day at school was spent trying to control her body and perform the requested tasks. Her brain was fatigued by the end of the day, and since she usually slept on the long bus ride home, her focus was better for homework. By waiting until later in the evening, she tended to struggle more, but the upside was Greg became more involved in helping her with homework. As they say, this was one of those situations where I needed to be wise and pick my battles.

The population of our quaint little town continued to grow, which resulted in the building of a new elementary school to accommodate the expansion. The old elementary school was then converted into a ninth-grade campus since it was conveniently located next door to the high school. Many parents were excited about this decision because before that the high school encompassed ninth grade to twelfth grade, and generally, there is a significant maturity difference between a ninth-grader and a tenth-grader. Another advantage to this new campus was that there was enough space in the building to move the Special Education Department over as well. The downside of this development was that the student growth changed the aide-to-student ratio. The aides would now have more than one student at a time, and as Rebecca's success in a regular classroom had been in large part due to her one-on-one time with an aide, I was fearful of what this would mean for her. In fact, this new protocol made me apprehensive enough that I felt compelled to request that Rebecca be pulled from the mainstream school and go strictly with Special Education.

While most parents fought hard, as I once did, to make sure their child was included in the regular classroom as much as possible, I was now requesting the opposite. Once again, I asked for a meeting with those who would be working with Rebecca and shared my desire to have her pulled. Talk about upsetting the apple cart! It reminded me of trying to get her released from the AEA years before with all the questions and forms I had to sign. My lobbying for exclusion was going against the norm, but my paramount motivation, as always, was to ensure that

Rebecca had the best education possible. I was not just asking for one year, but from that point forward because I believed it was imperative for her wellbeing. I was granted my request.

Rita, Rebecca's case manager, was a formidable match for her personality. After Reading and Math with Rita in the Life Skills classroom, Rebecca would then go to the Resource Room for English, History, and Health. Rita had a phenomenal ability to keep Rebecca on task, held her accountable, was consistent with communication, and worked well with the other teachers. It was impressive how easily she kept Rebecca stimulated in her academics, and we had a mutual expectation that Rebecca worked diligently toward reaching her potential. Our goal, as teacher and parent, was to provide Rebecca with our maximum support and the strategies necessary to facilitate a good outcome in school. Rita was almost a clone of Sheryl in her genuine enjoyment of working in the field of Special Education. She was motivated to see her students accomplish the skillset to learn regardless of their deficits. The paramount hurdle for all of us was Rebecca's lack of desire to perform the academic tasks she considered less desirable. She merely completed those assignments to appease the adults, but clearly was not giving them her all.

On the other hand, when Rebecca was interested in something, minimal effort was required to keep her focused or on task. This was a constant reminder to me that no matter how much we want something for our child, or anyone we care about, they must also want it for themselves if it is ever going to be of value. Rita and I were mindful of Rebecca's personality traits, and our strategy entailed pushing her until she began to shut down, which was our indication that the work was too complicated. In those situations, we eased up on our expectations and tried different approaches to teach the information so as not to overwhelm her. Our efforts kept Rebecca cooperative and focused on achieving the set goals.

It was once explained to me by a specialist that Rebecca's difficulty in reading was due to certain perimeters within her brain that were unable to comprehend some of the words and saw them as though in a different language. For this reason, any information being presented to Rebecca had to be visual or audial. Utilizing as many of her senses as possible would help her comprehend more of the material. Rebecca's IEP plan allowed for both a reduced workload and extra time to finish an assignment. This technique was beneficial in keeping her on task and reducing episodes of frustration, which resulted in more successes and forward movement rather than backsliding.

In the meantime our town continued its expansion, the latest addition being a brand-new sports club. Kathy, a community member who worked in water rehabilitation, approached the school with an interesting proposal. She wanted to start a Special Olympics swim team and was offering to coach any children who wanted to compete. In no time, kids, including Rebecca, were signing up, and the sports club kindly offered Kathy the use of the pool for training sessions. Thanks to Kathy's act of kindness, families not only had a new fun form of exercise, but were able to cultivate a beneficial support system for our special needs kids. It was truly a blessing for all of us.

The parents came together to pitch in, with some of the moms volunteering to help with the hands-on training of the team. As my work schedule didn't allow for that, Kathy instead utilized my secretarial skills. I used the information she provided to create a parents' newsletter, as well as a calendar and contact list for everyone. This allowed me to stay behind the scenes, where I do my best work.

The friendships formed through swimming quickly expanded to other activities, including birthday celebrations, picnics, and lunch and movie outings. Rebecca did an outstanding job of adhering to her diet, seamlessly working it into all her escapades with her Special Olympics teammates, even overnight sleepovers. She always carried a small backpack with her medication, food, wallet, and water, so I never had to worry about anything unless it was a new food or restaurant. Everyone was aware of her food restrictions and always accommodating to her needs, which was quite a big deal in the times before peanuts and other food allergies were so well-known.

It was inspiring to watch the kids develop and improve their social skills and experience personal growth through these activities. They took their training very seriously, a commitment that paid off when they went to State Competition, not once but multiple times! More importantly, they finally had another dimension to their lives other than being classmates in Special Education, where they were looked upon by their peers as misfits. For Rebecca, now fourteen, this was a game-changer. Sometimes her being mentally delayed complicated her perception of why other kids got invited to parties and, all too often, she did not. Having this new peer group lessened her sorrows, as they just naturally accepted one another without an ounce of discrimination regardless of the type and degree of their various disabilities. The transformation in her personality and maturity was encouraging, as was her excitement about having a boyfriend for the first time.

After witnessing the many blessings the swim team brought to these kids, I would never again doubt the profound difference one person can make in the lives of others. Kathy saw a need in our community and stepped forward to fill it, never imagining the beautiful ripple effect it would create. Her example motivated me to "pay it forward" and become more active in my church and more observant of others in general. Rather than just offering a smile or a simple hello, I now looked closer to see if perhaps they had a need.

Before we knew it Rebecca was ready to put yet another schoolyear behind her and enjoy the summer. Yolanda invited her to join 4-H with Jaci and asked a friend of hers to loan her an alpaca for Rebecca to work with and show at the fair. Each morning Rebecca would walk up the hill to Mark and Yolanda's house to groom and walk the alpaca and then brush their horses. She worked diligently with the alpaca to get it to walk beside her and follow her lead, and her efforts paid off when she showed at the fair and got a ribbon. Rebecca has always liked animals and enjoyed grooming the horses as much as riding with her aunt. My thoughts on horses are that they are beautiful and powerful animals that I admire from a distance.

The summer came to an end, and tenth grade awaited Rebecca's arrival. It seemed peculiar to be standing on the threshold of high school with Rebecca. How had the years passed so quickly? We had just celebrated Stephanie's graduation the year before and it seemed unbelievable that she had only been in the sixth grade when we moved to Washington.

Both sides of the family made the long trip to be part of the monumental occasion, an unruly Iowa posse that erupted in yells, whistles and tears as Stephanie walked proudly by in her cap and gown. She shined her brilliant smile our way and waved as she followed the line of graduates to their seats to await receiving their diplomas. For me and Greg it was a bittersweet moment because our mature and independent daughter planned to fly the nest shortly after graduation. She was moving out to live with friends, and though I felt it was too soon I knew I had to give her the space to embrace this next rite of passage. I also said plenty of extra prayers for her safety as she prepared to step out into the vast and sometimes scary world.

Now, as Rebecca prepared to enter high school, I also prayed that things would go as smoothly as possible. Though she had made tremendous progress, each schoolyear felt like trudging uphill toward the finish line. My emotions were all over the place, but Rebecca accepted this phase for what it was, another year of her being pushed by expectations from teachers and her mom. Starting tenth grade was not a huge emotional aspect in the scope of her world. It was just a new location and nothing more.

I tried to focus on the blessing that she was starting the year with the same teachers and the same placement and therefore, a smooth transition. Several weeks into the session, Rebecca was adapting well to the pace of high school while I kept glancing back over my shoulder as if a dark shadow was lurking in the distance. Since Rita had things under control and I no longer needed to be involved with the school scene, my sole responsibility was to help Rebecca with her homework. This was certainly encouraging, yet I also felt as though I was slacking in the parent department. After so many frantic years, our life finally seemed normal, or what one could consider normal with a teenage special needs daughter. It was an adjustment.

It was after the school year started that we decided to sell our home and buy an acre of land from Mark so Greg could fulfill his dream of designing and building a house. Since neither of us could physically build the house, we hired someone to do it for us using Greg's blueprints.

Mark and Greg cleared trees to make room for the house and put in the septic tank and drain field. Mark gave me a smaller chainsaw to help cut the tree trunks into rounds, which was not an easy or natural task for me. During one cut, the tree trunk snapped tight onto the chainsaw, jamming it inside. Mark eventually got it free but not before telling me I had been reassigned to wood hauling.

Our friend Kevin was kind enough to loan us his small two-bedroom trailer for the three of us to live while the house was being built. Greg had to take the front door off to get our side-by-side refrigerator inside, which left little room to maneuver through the kitchen nook. Rebecca's bedroom was on the left end of the trailer with a wall of closets, which we all shared. It was a tight fit for her double bed, so making the bed was a toss of the blanket up over the pillows.

Directly across from the front door was a closet-sized bathroom similar to the one in our first trailer, only this time there was no "big house" to go to when we wanted a bath. The kitchen nook was a tiny horseshoe area with a small stove, sink, and two stools to sit on. On the other side of the counter was the living room with Greg's recliner, a futon, and the TV against the wall to our bedroom that did not have a door. The room barely accommodated our queen size bed and a narrow table for our computer. We shared these extremely tight quarters for over a year, and it was quite impressive that the three of us survived the ordeal. When I say survived, it was not just close quarters with large personalities, but being engaged in a constant battle against the army of mice determined to share our humble tin abode.

The furnace did not work, and it had baseboard heat, which left the metal ductwork under the floors as a sort of rodent transit system. You could hear them scurrying back and forth, so I filled every crack with that expanding foam to prevent infiltration into our living quarters. As we had one of the very few cats that were actually scared of mice, we had to rely on a trap to keep them at bay. Greg was in charge of setting and placing the mousetrap down into the vent of the bathroom floor as well as disposal. Those critters multiplied like rabbits, and it may sound cruel, but it was a relief to hear the snap of the trap from their continuous attempt at invading our space. The extermination process declined but never ceased the entire time we lived in that metal residence. Finally, the big day arrived, and we moved into our three-bedroom home with a daylight basement that we planned to convert into living quarters for Rebecca when we could afford it.

You know that saying, "If you build it, they will come?" Well, shortly after we moved into the house Stephanie decided that perhaps she had moved out too early. She was finding it difficult to work and attend classes at college, where she was training to be a medical assistant, so she returned home to save money. She would try again later for independence, and for now it was just nice having our family back under one roof.

The beginning of eleventh grade was as seamless as the year before, and everything appeared satisfactory on Rebecca's IEP plan. In fact, in addition to her academic goals she now had an additional protocol for job skills training, both on and off campus. With guidance from a life skills coach, she and other students who were mentally and physically able were transported from school to volunteer at local businesses. Rebecca was taken to a local grocery store to dust shelves, and I was notified that she was not cooperative with this task. Since I was unaware that dusting was one of the skills she would be learning I had not apprised them of her allergy to dust. After that they placed her with other classmates on campus to make dog bones and package them to sell, which was a perfect solution since she liked to bake.

Things seemed to be back on track until Rebecca came home after school and told me she had been shoved by a girl while walking in the hall. She said she had not done or said anything to this girl to warrant this aggression. I contacted Rita, who said she had not been aware of the problem but would now make inquiries as to what was going on between the two. An aide from the classroom told Rita that she had seen Rebecca using her two index fingers to make a sign of the cross when the other girl walked by and felt that this was an act of antagonism on Rebecca's part. When Rebecca got home, I asked her why she did that, and she said the girl was being mean and saying bad things to her when she was walking alone. I told her that I would make an appointment with the guidance counselor but in the meantime, she should stop engaging in any way with this girl and find a different way to get to class.

When we met with the counselor he told Rebecca to ignore this girl's taunts and that would most likely resolve the problem. He was wrong, and I soon found myself back in his office, this time because the girl had bounced Rebecca off a vending machine. The counselor quickly explained that the school had called the mother and left a message, but she had yet to respond.

Appalled, I told him the lack of immediate action regarding an assault on my daughter was both negligent and unacceptable. His reply was to share that before the attack he had seen this girl stomping around in what was clearly an agitated state. He even admitted to wondering why she was not in class. *What?!* This supposed professional had witnessed a student in a rage, acting out, and skipping class, and he had done nothing! By that point I was also in a rage, and no one – certainly not this person – would be able to talk me down. I spun around and stormed out, my next destination the local police department. My intention was to file a restraining order against this bully, but after hearing the circumstances the officer informed me that they preferred to let the school handle "minor" problems such as this. *Hello?* Was I just knocked back to Mayberry? (For those of you too young to remember, Mayberry was the fictional small (and backwards) town in the 1960s show Mayberry R.F.D. You can google it.) It seemed so, but Sherriff Andy Taylor was nowhere to be found, Deputy Barney Fife was absolutely no help, and my blood pressure was still on the rise. To avoid going to jail myself for assault, I decided to retreat to fight another day.

When Greg got home from work, I was still pacing and he had a difficult time calming me down. We needed to be thankful that the outcome had not been worse for Rebecca and figure out what our options were regarding the situation. By the next morning, the school called to notify me that an adult would be with Rebecca anytime she was out of class. I suspected that there was a "hotline" between the local police department and the school, and they knew I had attempted to seek legal involvement. At least I had their attention, and the staff gave me a wide berth after that, other than Rita, who never changed her demeanor. Stephanie later told me that she had a friend still in the school who'd made it very clear to the bully that she had better not talk bad or touch Rebecca again.

Senior year was now upon us, but Rebecca would not be graduating because she lacked full credits. The tradition in Special Education was for seniors without enough credits to put on their caps and gowns and walk with their senior class anyway. While I respected their wanting to participate in this milestone, I did not agree with it for Rebecca. This ceremony was not supposed to be a dress rehearsal, but a moment to honor all the hard work she had put into her education. When Greg and I told her our wish was that she attain all the necessary credits before putting on the cap and gown, Rebecca was disappointed about not walking with her classmates but understood that we just wanted it to be the real deal.

Special Education students remain in the school system until the age of twenty-one, when they transition out. Rebecca's next three years of school were focused on achieving the necessary grades for graduation and learning life skills to ensure that she could be as self-sufficient as possible once she exited the program. Shelley, a particularly creative teacher in Life Skills, started an "Eats Café." One day a week, school staff would come into the class for breakfast. The menu had simple foods like pancakes, breakfast burritos, scrambled eggs, juice, coffee, and milk. Students took turns cooking, taking orders, clearing tables, and cleaning up. What began as an in-house pilot program was such a success that they decided to open it up to our local community. It is still going strong today.

The Special Olympic swim team was still thriving as well, and the time had come for Kathy to pass the coaching torch to someone else. Several parents stepped up to take over the responsibilities and did a tremendous job, while other parents branched out to incorporate a bowling team. Students who had no interest in swimming were excited to join the bowling team, as were many swimmers. The kids now had two different Special Olympic events to participate in, and I was both surprised and pleased to see Rebecca become so active in sports at that stage of her life. She was so passionate about her swimming and bowling that we had to buy her an awards board for all her medals and ribbons! The motto of Special Olympics is, "Let me win, but if I can't win, let me be brave in the attempt." Our slogan for Rebecca was that the competitions were first and foremost about the fun; if it became only about the prize, she had the wrong attitude.

One of the paramount advantages of living in this community is how sincerely they embrace and support special needs kids and young adults. As they navigate life they are rarely if ever treated unkindly or bullied, something neither they nor their parents take for granted. Our local fire department acknowledged the Special Olympic sports by inviting the various teams to ride in the fire engines and inside the rescue boat during town parades. Rebecca had an opportunity to cross riding in a limousine off her bucket list when she and her teammates took one to an awards dinner. One of the coaches had connections with the limo's owner and arranged this fantastic surprise, and the tearful parents stood in line, taking pictures. The athletes were laughing and beaming with so much joy as they climbed inside, and we were extremely thankful to have such generous people in our kids' lives.

After just a one-year delay, Rebecca officially donned her red cap and gown with the white sash and joined the graduating class of 2003. She welcomed the tradition of having her senior picture taken and our Iowa family once again traveled the long distance to witness her extraordinary moment. It had taken thirteen years of consistent hard work to get her to this moment of triumph, and even as I overflowed with pride for her, I acknowledged that this never would have happened without the countless people who assisted her in the long, challenging journey. My wish was that those who believed she could not be a functioning member of society, let alone graduate, could see her at that moment. What if I had accepted wholeheartedly those experts' philosophies about Rebecca's limitations in life? Thankfully, I had the wisdom of people like Mike, who reminded me all those years earlier that these experts do not have all the answers and are simply going by whatever the standard test is at the time. His words kept me focused not on what was "impossible," but what I could do and needed to do to help Rebecca adapt to her deficits and reach her full potential.

Once Rebecca had tasted the victory of graduation, she tried to convince us that she was ready to leave the program, but we held firm and insisted she waited until she was twenty-one. Although she had achieved the grades necessary to graduate, she still lacked the essential skills to adapt to a working environment; she also needed to work on developing people skills. To help her have a better understanding of these concepts, I "hired" her to perform several jobs around the house that were usually my responsibility. Once we had a set of tasks, we settled on a pay scale, and I reminded her that this process was like in the real world - I was her boss and would hold her accountable. If I had to tell her more than once to do the work she would get a reduction in pay, and if I were unhappy with her performance she would have to redo the job without any additional compensation.

As with anything asked of Rebecca, there were struggles and successes, which I accepted as part of the never-ending learning curve. Her income covered the cost of her going to the movies or out to eat with her friends, and we continued working on creating a budget.

The next two years were about the same, with Rebecca putting in her time in the program with little to no negative feedback from the school. We relished the break from academic struggles and embraced a period of relative tranquility. Then, in what felt like the blink of an eye Rebecca turned twenty-one. It was time to transition out of school, another joyous milestone that also carried with it a rather significant consequence. Leaving school meant she no longer qualified for Greg's health insurance, and her seizures, medications, and frequent blood monitoring tests were beyond our financial means. Thus began the arduous process of applying for government disability coverage, with all its appointments, evaluations, and seemingly endless forms to fill out. I was fearful that she would be denied, but we had documentation of her mental delay from medical professionals and school districts that dated back to her infancy.

The meeting with the government physiologist reminded me of our first encounter with the AEA - Rebecca was evaluated, then the two of us spoke to the psychologist, then I went in alone. The difference this time was that Rebecca was aware of why the evaluation was being done and asked questions I had not had to deal with the first time around. While we waited to hear whether she qualified for medical and financial assistance, I focused on teaching her how to make and keep a budget. Rebecca was proficient at counting money and quickly picked up on how to write and deduct checks. Our next exercise was to go shopping. While she checked out I stood off to the side, waiting to help if needed. She understood that she needed to know how to count money, not only so she could conduct the daily business of living, but so she would not be a victim of a dishonest person who may try to shortchange her.

It was while making a shopping list that Rebecca leveled one of the biggest shocks of my life. Now that she was twenty-one and no longer in school, she planned to kick the diet to the curb. I was completely flabbergasted. Why, after seventeen years of healthy eating, would she want to put unhealthy foods into her clean body?

I automatically said, "absolutely not," and was promptly hit with a reality check. Rebecca had the right to make that decision as an adult. Greg and I did have power of attorney for medical and financial issues, but that was more of an emergency measure. Otherwise, she had a right to her independence just like any other grown woman. Still, my heart began doing that tug-of-war thing again. Flashbacks of what she was like before the diet began spinning in my mind. What if she became aggressive again? She was not a four-year-old anymore, and at almost six feet tall, she could definitely kick my butt.

I agreed to let her try it, but she needed to accept that if her behavior became a problem, she would go back on the diet. Her mood was somewhat altered with the change in food but not drastically, and she seemed to manage the noticeable difference that came from eating colored and artificial foods. It was disappointing to me that she had given up eating the healthy way, but I was encouraged that all those years of behavior modifications had made a difference. Within months of eating all manner of things, she did, as many of us would, gain weight, but when I asked her if she felt the old side effects like headaches had returned, she said no. I couldn't help but wonder if her seizure medication had something to do with her not having those symptoms.

Suddenly, Rebecca's world had become one of culinary delights. As she sampled all the forbidden foods she had desired while on the diet, I was even more amazed by her ability to stay true to the restrictions for all those years. I think the most comical thing was when she ate a store-bought birthday cake. As she delighted in the sugary treat, she told me she did not want to hurt my feelings but all those birthday cakes I made from scratch were dense and not that good. Laughing, I asked what else she choked down to be polite and bless her heart she said she liked most of what I made. Then, with that devilish grin of hers, she admitted that she had always hated my meatloaf! I agreed that I hated it too and only made it because her dad and Stephanie liked it.

CHAPTER NINE

Life after High School

"As much as you may want to curse your challenges, instead simply regard them as invitations to demonstrate your courage."

Margie Warrell

By the time Rebecca transitioned out of school she had already been employed part-time as a dishwasher at the local senior living complex for one year. Eventually she learned food prep as well, but what she loved most about the job was meeting the residents who eventually became like adoptive family. Frank was her favorite because he was a fun character and usually had a new joke to tell her each week.

We also got a government directory of agencies that help individuals with disabilities once they transition out of school. Once again, I was back in the trenches as a foot soldier and advocate for Rebecca in maneuvering through the multiple services. Some of the benefits helped people find job coaches and tutors; attain further education; and locate designated financial payees. After reading through the pamphlets, I decided to wait on that daunting phase until it was necessary. Rebecca was already employed and socially active; life was finally uncomplicated, and I just wanted a break.

Due to Rebecca's seizure disorder, she would never have the privilege of driving, so we provided her transportation unless she took the bus or rode with friends. Living on Camano Island was beautiful, but there was only one way on and off, and fortunately, the county provided Community Transit bus service. Rebecca took the bus to work since her shift started after I had already left for my job. She only worked a couple of days a week but always got down the hill from our house in time to catch the bus and adapted amazingly well to reading bus schedules and maneuvering about town on another bus line. Sometimes after work, she walked downtown to hang out before showing up to ride home with me. Our parent support group was an invaluable asset and allowed us working moms the flexibility to fulfill our obligations for transportation on the weekends.

With Rebecca no longer in school, her social interactions were much more limited, and other than birthday parties or sporting events, she was more isolated compared to her former classmates who lived in town. Worried about her being alone so much, I asked around to see how other parents were handling life without the structure of school. Our lives now revolved around full-time responsibility for our adult offspring, who had gone from being at school five days a week to wandering around the house in need of activities to keep them busy. I was told about this event being hosted by the Disability Act Program where a young man was giving a free presentation and interviews to special needs young adults. (I don't remember this young man's name so to make things less confusing I will call him "Adam.")

When I walked into the presentation I saw two of Rebecca's former classmates and their moms there as well. Once everyone had settled in, Adam explained that he would be helping each of them create a Life Map, which would be formed later from the information they provided that day. He propped a large white paper tablet upon an easel and called on the only boy as his first volunteer. Adam asked the boy to name five things he wanted to accomplish in his life, and my attention drifted toward Rebecca as I wondered what she would share on her turn. Adam wrote down the five things across the paper and drew a big circle around each word; he then asked the boy to name several actions for each one of the words. As he wrote these down, he explained to the boy that these actions would now be the necessary steps for him to follow in order to accomplish each goal. Adam made it sound so darn simple.

While the rest of us watched, listened, and waited for the next person's turn, Rebecca leaned over and whispered that she did not want to participate because it would be embarrassing. As if Adam suspected what she was saying to me, he called on her next. When she told him she was not interested, he gently encouraged her to try. Finally she agreed, and as I looked on I was very impressed with how effortlessly he connected with her. Just as he had with the boy, Adam used a calm tone of voice while giving her his full attention throughout the interaction. I was amazed at how quickly he got Rebecca to share, without hesitation, her deep inner thoughts. A few things she divulged were a revelation to me and made me think perhaps I did not know her as thoroughly as I thought. Truly, this man had a gift.

I was not surprised that her first goal was to live on her own since she often expressed that desire. The steps she named for that goal were getting a full-time job, finding an apartment, living in town for better access to bus transportation, and learning how to cook better. Her second goal, again no surprise, was to have the ability to drive, which was not realistic. The third goal was to meet her favorite race car driver Kasey Kane, which she later achieved by calling a radio station that was giving away tickets to see him in his hometown. Her fourth goal was to ride in a limo, which as mentioned earlier she also accomplished, this by being part of the Special Olympics. The fifth goal was the one that broke my heart: she wanted to find a way to fix her brain. I'd had no idea how deeply it bothered and frustrated her to have limitations, and hearing her share that reminded me of the doctor who had qualified her for the disability benefits. He had expressed how sad and unfortunate it was that Rebecca was smart enough to realize that she had permanent mental delays. His insight had not truly registered with me then, but it did on that day.

Once Adam finished up with the kids he gave each of us moms some one-on-one time, and I found his insights extremely helpful. He asked what our long-term expectations were for Rebecca, and I stated that we hoped one day for her to live independently. I told him about us having the house built and that we had dedicated half of the daylight basement to make into a one-bedroom apartment for her. Adam was silent for a moment, then asked if I was interested in his input regarding the apartment idea, which I was. He highly suggested that we might want to reconsider this type of setup for Rebecca, if our hope was truly for her it live independently. Living attached to our home, he said, might lead to greater dependency and ultimately inhibit her from adapting to living on her own.

Adam proposed that we instead consider making the space into a large bedroom and not put in a kitchenette or bathroom as planned. By her having to go upstairs, to use the bathroom and prepare meals, it would keep her in the family routine while giving her a quiet living space. Greg agreed with Adam's assessment, and instead of putting up walls, he built a closet in the area under the stairs. We divided the room in half, and the section by the exterior door and one of the windows would be her living room with the futon, area rug, and her TV cabinet. The other half, by the second window, became her bedroom area with an interior door leading to the stairs. Greg installed a second handrail to accommodate Rebecca's depth perception problem and provide her stability. We carpeted the stairs as well. Rebecca helped seal the concrete floors and picked a navy-blue color to paint the walls. She was thrilled with her own space and immediately posted a "Knock First" sign on her door to let visitors know they needed permission to enter.

Rebecca was now responsible for preparing her meals during the week, and I cooked for the three of us on the weekends. She learned how to make a meal plan, a grocery list, and was getting much better at budgeting. Her independence was encouraging, so my next objective was to teach her how to run the washer and dryer and be responsible for her laundry. Yes, I can hear you thinking that she should have acquired this essential skill long before now! The fault is absolutely mine because of my dominant personality for wanting things done a particular way. Rebecca was accepting these responsibilities and without an attitude, which was a blessing.

The day Rebecca received her Life Map in the mail was a fun one. Adam and his colleagues had really outdone themselves, creating an impressive piece of work that included an adorable caricature of her smiling face off to the side of her goals and steps. The artist who had drawn the map used bright colors on a large white poster size sheet of glossy paper. There were five puffy clouds, each with a drawing inside that represented one of the five goals – in Rebecca's case, an apartment, automobile, racecar, limo, and books for learning. Below each cloud, the steps for reaching that goal were listed in separate balloons. All Rebecca had to do was start at the bottom balloon and work her way up toward her goal. Whenever we unrolled her colorful map and gazed upon all her possibilities, I couldn't deny that creating that map had a substantial impact not only on Rebecca, but on us as well. Greg and I were especially grateful to Adam for his advice about how we could help Rebecca have her own private living space without hindering her ultimate goal of living on her own.

Our lives fell into an effortless rhythm of jobs, chores, and solely moving from one day to the next. We did not miss the constant apprehension, struggles, frustrations, or expectations of the last eighteen years of school. Rebecca adjusted well to life without classrooms, but it created obstacles for me as I maneuvered as best as I could being in the teacher's seat without insight or assistance. How was I supposed to respond to whatever the future decided to drop next into my lap? There was always a next in my world! I was flying solo for the first time since Rebecca was in preschool. Although my family and friends were supportive, there was no way they could ever truly comprehend the depth of emotions and circumstances that raising a special needs individual entails. The support from school was gone, and I was awkwardly stumbling along.

The turmoil and isolation from any disorder automatically enrolls you as a member of the undesirable parent club. If I had the power, I would permanently nail shut that door to protect others from the gut-wrenching pain of being powerless to alleviate what life has inflicted upon your child. I was hijacked as a participant in this heartless club, and it took years of anger, and frustration before I could see the clarity that Rebecca's life was a blessing. All the other stuff was undeniably hardships, but no amount of angry fist-shaking, or cursing would ever compare to the pain of a parent whose child would never be able to see, hear, speak, or walk. Once I embraced that perception, the adversities in my life seemed less traumatic and allowed me to focus more on how Rebecca was blooming and growing toward a more independent young woman. From her milestones, a different set of challenges developed, which basically meant that I needed to find a different method of adapting to whatever arose from that change.

A pattern started emerging after Rebecca turned twenty-one, one in which she would focus only on her chronological age and expect to have all the things typically associated with that age. In truth, the concept that there was a difference between her mental capacity and her actual age was one Rebecca had never accepted entirely; however, now that distinction seemed to fade even further.

"I am twenty-one," she'd say, "a legal adult, and you cannot tell me what to do anymore!"

This became her mantra for each birthday, as I continued to try and tenderly explain that some facets of her birth age were still beyond that of her mental capabilities. I always tried to be respectful, compassionate, and never cruel or bitchy in my explanations regarding her deficits because it was a painful subject for me as well. Yet this time no matter how carefully I chose my words I seemed to be unable to make an impact.

After four years of this ongoing argument, I became exhausted trying to be patient with her, and instead of gentleness, she finally got the reality. On her twenty-fifth birthday, I bluntly stated that it mattered not if she was twenty-five or fifty years old, her brain would never be more mature than that of a teenager. It was excruciating to be that honest, but nothing had worked thus far to get her to understand that what she wanted with each birthday was most likely forever beyond her grasp. To prevent her from experiencing total devastation, I quickly reassured her that I was confident that she would continue to learn new things, but she needed to let go of the expectations of having all the amenities that came with certain ages. The validation that I finally got through was in not having the conversation again, but I am a realist and understand that Rebecca will never reach the point where she will outgrow the need for my intervention.

Life is ever-changing, and the news was reporting it, we began feeling it, and companies started laying off people. The economy was moving in the wrong direction and Rebecca, along with several of her classmates, was the first to lose their jobs. This of course had an immense impact upon them, not just because of the loss of money but their routine as well. They had nowhere to go or something to look forward to each week. Their jobs were more of a social aspect than a work environment. Our small-town businesses had no choice but to have the first causalities be those with special needs to ensure that the elders, husbands, wives, and young adults would not lose their family income. Rebecca handled the loss of her job with grace and understood that it was not due to her lack of performance but the lousy economy. To her, it was just life, and her ability to accept situations and not fret about it readily was her natural gift. She never wasted too much time or energy stressing over things, and I sure envied her that ability.

When the economy started recovering Rebecca courageously walked into several retailers asking if they were hiring. Even though there were no opportunities available, she just kept trying with the expectation that one day she would find a job. Her persistence paid off when she got a dishwashing job at a local restaurant, which made Greg and I wonder if she was ready for the next step. I began checking in town for a facility that accommodated adults with disabilities, and the only one had a two-year wait list, so I filled out an application. Every day on my way to work, I drove past a housing complex for Senior Living down the street from work and always thought it would be the perfect setting for Rebecca. She adored the elderly and being a higher-functioning adult with mental challenges; she would be an asset within that community. I talked with the manager and learned that the complex only had a couple of designated apartments with government rent assist - none of them currently available.

Still, after I told her a bit about Rebecca she let me fill out an application to send to corporate for approval. While we waited to hear back, two of our friends happened to move into the complex and offered to endorse Rebecca as a tenant. In several months she was approved as a tenant, but that apartment was not government-rent assist, so she moved in while Greg and I paid the subsidy until government assistance became available. We had to provide a notarized letter stating that we would be responsible for her rent if she did not pay and for any damages. By the age of twenty-nine, Rebecca had reached her first goal on her life map and was living independently, and fortunately, the government rent assistance was available before the end of the year. She was ecstatic to be on her own and proud of the hard work that enabled her this opportunity.

Again, I wished that those who did not believe in her could see her achieve another milestone in life and that she was a productive member of society. My wish was not with the intent to rub her accomplishments in their faces, but hopefully, enlighten them to the potential of these kids; I want them to see possibilities rather than limitations. Rebecca's success was because I never gave up, always believed there was a plan, sought out people to help me attain knowledge, and learned the skills necessary to help Rebecca reach her potential. I trusted my gut, followed my instincts, and became a sponge when information was available. That tenacity kept me focused on whatever it took to help Rebecca, and not once did I consider that she would not be a functioning member of society. My fierce determination was fueled by the belief it was my responsibility and obligation as her parent.

More parents became involved in Special Olympics, which eventually included a soccer team and a basketball team. Rebecca joined these two new teams as well as the Kiwanis sponsored Aktion Club in town. The Aktion Club began with the Kiwanis Organization in 1988 and led by George D. Swartout in Florida for adults with disabilities. The club became an official "Service Leadership Program of the Kiwanis International" in October of 2000 and included the United States, Canada, Australia, Philippines, Jamaica, Bahamas, and Malaysia. In her group, Rebecca has held the office of Treasurer and Secretary, and they do service work by helping with the Kiwanis fish fries as well as working with the State of Washington E-Cycle program by collecting computers, monitors, and TVs on the first Saturday of the month.

This local organization is also active in putting together different dances and other events to gather adults from our town and the surrounding communities. They provide the young adults an opportunity to mingle, have fun, and develop friendships outside of their tight circles. Rebecca is also involved with volunteering at the Warm Beach Christian Community for the month of July as a caregiver during the Special Needs Camp. Then she goes directly from there to get the local fair grounds ready for the three-day fair and gets free entrance in exchange for her help. She also volunteers again after Thanksgiving at the Warm Beach Christian Community every winter as they present the Lights of Christmas, which is a big event for the Puget Sound area. These annual events are the highlight of her summer and fall activities and have made her relatively well known among our community.

We still face issues with our strong-willed and stubborn daughter who seems to always want to control situations and people. One might say she is somewhat "bossy" and when one of her peers or a mom approaches me to express irritation with Rebecca for something she has said or done, my auto response is for them to talk to her. Having them address her directly makes her accountable and has more impact than if it comes from me. The days of me being responsible for Rebecca's actions are over; she lives on her own and is an adult. Her personality is what it is, and no amount of effort on my part, or anyone else's, has been able to correct that character trait. There tends to be unrest among

Rebecca and her peer group, and I once again think back to the words of that psychologist. Rebecca functions at a higher level than many with mental disabilities, is more mature, and lives on her own while managing her finances; therefore I think she is more likely to be frustrated when she feels hindered by her limitations.

I do monitor Rebecca's finances to make sure she pays her bills on time and stays within her budget and would love to say that life is finally stress-free, but that would not be honest. Even without disabilities, adult offspring can have issues in which a parent needs to become involved, whether they like it or not. Rebecca continues to adapt and learn, and I am still uncertain as to what exactly her ultimate potential is; in the meantime I just remain alert and continue to be her safety net. She teaches me things from time to time and has this remarkable sense of direction while I am forever turned around and confused. I take a left when it should be a right, and Rebecca makes an excellent navigator. She has a wickedly funny sense of humor, sees a need long before anyone else, and has great compassion for strangers. Sometimes our family would appreciate her being as compassionate and patient with us as she tends to be with others, but such is life.

My best guess as to why Rebecca is not as patient with us is because she sees us as the "hounding forces" whose primary objective is to tell her how to live her life. She is hellbent on making us understand that she is in charge of her life, and rightly so if Rebecca had the true mental capacity of a thirty-five-year-old woman. Unfortunately, her maturity equivalent is still that of an angry teenager fighting for independence. Sometimes trying to reason with her is reminiscent of when she was a child and would not come down from the slide and only my threat of coming up after her would get her to comply. Greg seems to be waiting for the magic light bulb to go on and make all the struggles disappear, but even the Wizard of Oz has no remedy to fix that for Rebecca.

In the five years that Rebecca has lived in her apartment we have had to deal with a few issues regarding overdrafts, which unfortunately led to us showing up at her door. Both of us would prefer to walk on a bed of nails than address money issues or remind her to keep a tidy apartment. Our spitfire daughter takes the stance that we obtain pleasure from sticking our noses into her business and disputes accountability with an abundance of excuses. Since I have always been the hands-on parent, my job is to take the lead and remind her that we did nothing wrong and she is responsible for the consequences for her actions. Greg watches and listens, hoping he does not have to become the drill sergeant and bellow at our agitated daughter to calm down as she fidgets and no doubt wishes she could kick my butt (which she could most certainly do since acquiring a black belt in Taekwondo). Thankfully, Rebecca is not physically aggressive and loves me enough to walk away before she disassembles me. Coincidentally, taking Taekwondo did help tremendously to curb her short fuse, and she has never attempted to inflict physical assault on anyone, well, not since grade school when she knocked the heads of those two mean little girls together!

Rebecca grasps the importance of using her words when exasperated and is aware that she must never lose her self-control and cross that line. She took to heart the words of wisdom I gave her a long time ago in that she could think all manner of things inside her head but is accountable for what comes out of her mouth. Rarely does Rebecca get that angry and when she is having a hissy fit, I am usually the one to absorb the verbal blast. When she was little, a psychologist told her to crumple up paper and bounce it off the walls to release her frustrations and then clean up after. That worked for a while, but of course the emotions of puberty were not as easily released with paper wads, so I gave her permission to vent with me and promised never to hold a grudge, retaliate, or stop loving her.

One day Rebecca came over to the house to tell me about an issue she had at work with one of the managers. The man told her to clean the grease off the kitchen wall by the griddle since she was not busy washing dishes, so she washed as far as she could reach and returned to her dishwashing duties. He snapped at Rebecca that she had not finished the job of cleaning the grease off the higher part of the wall and told her to get a step ladder and finish. She tried to explain to him about her inability to be on a ladder due to a problem with her depth perception, but he just angrily yelled at her to leave. When she returned for her shift the next day, he was still hostile, so she quit. I felt that she correctly handled the situation by trying to explain her reason to the manager and proud of her for standing up for herself. The momma bear in me wanted to go to that man and ask him why he refused to respect her inability to be on a ladder.

The place also had a female manager, and whenever I encountered her she always told me how much she enjoyed having Rebecca work there. Perhaps this man did not have the same experience; perhaps he was just not nice. Whatever the case, I fought the urge to stick my nose in her business and was proud that Rebecca did not come running to me to fight her battle. She had handled the situation successfully all on her own. It showed good decision-making skills and demonstrated that she was acquiring more life skills to help her function in the adult world. However, that altercation with the manager did affect Rebecca's confidence, and she postponed looking for work. I gave her some time to process the situation and then suggested she consider doing some volunteer work. It concerned me that she had started isolating herself by staying in her apartment.

One Sunday after Mass, Rita, her teacher from high school, asked Rebecca if she would consider coming to talk to the current class about life after school. Rita felt Rebecca's success in getting jobs and living on her own could help some of the students. Rebecca told her she would think about it and let her know. I expressed what an honor it was that Rita had asked, and how sharing her story could give hope to the kids still in the program. As they say, the nut does not fall far from the tree, and as Rebecca shares my discomfort with standing up in front of people and speaking she declined the invitation. She did, however, start looking for jobs again. I am not sure if Rita asking her to speak was the push Rebecca needed, but she got her confidence back, as well as a job at Jack in the Box, a fast food chain, cleaning the lobby, restrooms, breaking down boxes, and putting away stock. Her ability to fearlessly walk into a business and ask for a job is inspiring to me, especially since my courage has never been that strong when it comes to pounding the pavement for work.

What I have come to understand, which is both frustrating and inspiring, is that Rebecca can be tenacious, confident, and motivated when it comes to something she wants. She is truly comfortable with who she is and does not care at all what others think about her, her sense of fashion, or the numerous bold hair colors she has chosen. Sometimes I do wonder if her self-assured attitude was cultivated as a result of the unkind words and actions of other kids during her childhood. Each time she came crying to me because someone called her a name or she was harassed, I would explain that mean kids are unhappy, need our prayers, and not to be like them. Happy people spread kindness, angry people spread pain and unhappiness, and that I hoped she would never make someone feel as bad as she was feeling at that moment. This explanation was my version of "Sticks and Stones can break your bones, but words can never hurt you!"

The hell they don't!

When my parents responded with that old-time saying for getting over hurt feelings, it never gave me much comfort or any understanding as to why I was picked on or hit by other kids. While growing up, the motto in our home was that we were to buck it up, dry our tears, go out and play, and stop reacting. There was pride in being tough and shame in being a crybaby or sissy. I was just thankful that Rebecca did not allow that pain to make her a mean person. The reality is that we all experience hills and valleys – both milestones and bumps in the road. Looking back at the roads Rebecca and I have traveled, I appreciate how far we have come and believe that whatever life brings our way we will prevail. Quitting or just sliding through has never been part of our personalities, and I sincerely thank the Lord for that. Growth comes from struggles, and I am a better person and parent because of this journey with Rebecca. Would I have preferred a more comfortable and peaceful passage such as the one I had with Stephanie? Of course! However, each of my daughters has taught me things, brought me much joy and love, and certainly enhanced my potential to be a better person.

By the end of summer there was less business at the Jack in the Box and they cut Rebecca's hours; then she lost the job. She decided to take some time off because she did not want a new job to interfere with her stint at the Lights of Christmas. The first couple of years she worked this event she was in a costume and greeted the children, but then was elevated to the position of helping direct cars for parking. Because she was a dedicated volunteer, they provided her accommodations as well as an evening meal and breakfast. I would drop her off at the facility since it was outside of town and then pick her up the next day. She looked forward to doing this each year, and still does. Our little social butterfly has spread her wings and developed roots in town, making many friends, and as a parent of a special needs' adult, I could not ask for a better community to call home.

After the holidays, Rebecca found herself missing the social interaction of a working environment, so she applied – and was hired - at Mc Donald's. Frank, the manager, sees her potential and has taught her to operate the fryers and take food out to waiting cars, as well as some other jobs. She loves being trusted to learn different skills other than just clean and stock. Rebecca does not have the skills to take orders or run the cash register, but it is impressive that she has gotten into the kitchen area to perform tasks. With each accomplishment I've watched her stand taller with confidence for what she had learned to do on her own. Observing Rebecca maneuver through life has helped me believe she will manage okay when I am no longer here to be her safety net. I know Stephanie will watch over her, but we found a lawyer who specializes in disabilities to protect Rebecca.

Rebecca is my hero because after all she has endured, not once has she asked, "Why me?" I am also in awe of her ability to figure out the latest technology; indeed, she has often been my teacher with regard to these things. When I was first learning to use a computer, Rebecca would rearrange the icons on my desktop and then laugh hysterically at my frustration of trying to put them back where they belonged. It makes me wonder how today she can read manuals and comprehend the information when she struggled with reading in school. It is insights like these that support my belief she is still able to process and learn things that have absolutely nothing to do with the delay in her maturity capacity. Rebecca is just a big kid with a huge heart who loves games, fairs, music, movies, sports, and life in general. She has developed from a child with so many struggles into a confident young woman who sees the world through a different lens than most people. The saying, "No guts no glory" describes her as she faces situations with courage, confidence, and lives, life on her terms.

CHAPTER TEN

Looking Back at Our Love Story

"Parents give us a strong foundation of values in which to build our life, and each of us has to be the architect of the finished product. After all; we are all under construction during this life, building, changing, and sometimes tearing down parts of the framework that constitutes who we are."

Doug Crimmins

Looking back, I certainly never anticipated that my life would involve such intense twists and turns that I would need to maneuver and overcome. It is obvious now, at this stage of my life, that the struggles I encountered and withstood were necessary to mold the young woman of my youth into the resilient person I am today. Surely, the difficulties I faced over the years gave me the strength I needed while striving to be the best wife possible. My determination to make my marriage work nurtured my ability to acquire patience and maturity, which were key to adapting to the role of motherhood. I honestly believe that my desire to cultivate a comfortable and flexible relationship with Greg enhanced my ability to face the challenging components of parenting Rebecca.

At this point in the story, you might be thinking that Greg and I were merely fortunate to have managed and survived the turbulence in our lives, but that would be a misconception. It was through enduring those numerous ordeals that motivated our maturity and ultimately built our character. We were not totally naive or particularly immature when we got married, but we still had a long way yet to go to evolve into who we are today. Like most young girls, I grew up dreaming about the day my knight in shining armor would whisk me away, get married, and live happily ever after, and life would be easy-peasy. I guess I did meet my knight in shining armor, we did get married, and ultimately, we are living happily ever after. It just did not happen as I had envisioned. What I discovered is that having a stable relationship allowed us to get through life's ups and downs, and I want to share with you the love story that started it all.

Growing up, I lacked self-confidence, suffered from extreme anxiety, and rarely strayed far from the safety of my family. As a teenager, I preferred to blend into the background of social events. It was hard for me to silence the pain of never feeling comfortable in my own skin, and I never felt good enough unless I had my glass of liquid courage. My drinking was not problematic, at first. After all, it was the same behavior exhibited by my parents, extended family, and friends. In time, I would learn that alcohol was not my friend.

After graduating high school, in 1974, I got a job working as a checker for Safeway Grocery where it was a man's world and necessitated having a thick skin. I had to endure intense training for several weeks at forty hours per week to learn how to ring up each item, by hand, according to the department, and then by price. Oh, how I would have loved to be of this generation with scanners! When I passed the accuracy and speed test for checking my feet barely touched the ground as I did a happy dance for my accomplishments. While developing the necessary skills to be a checker, I discovered a fascinating element about myself that I had never observed before. It was easier for me to learn using visual and physical techniques than it was by reading and, looking back now, I realize that Rebecca learns a lot like her momma.

The anxieties on my first day of work faded quickly when the manager apprised me that I would not be checking but bagging groceries and carrying them out for the customer. Yep, back then, the groceries were bagged and taken to the car to be loaded! During my training, no one had explained to me that I would be starting at the bottom and had to earn my position as a checker. My initial reaction was to say, "Go to hell" and walk out the door. But this was my first reality check in the adult working world. Life was still not fair! Somehow, I had believed that working in a full-time setting would inevitably offer me protection from that disturbing fact of life. Since I needed the job, I plastered a smile on my face and fumed on the inside while making sure not to break any of the customer's eggs. During lunch, I vented to a friend who had worked there for several years, since high school, and she explained why I was starting at the bottom.

The department manager believed having all newly hired checkers start as baggers gave them a vital understanding and respect for that job and the person. Although I did not appreciate it at the time, it was an effective way of learning that lesson and one I never forgot. Just the same, it still would have been considerate to be forewarned in training, because what if my Irish mouth had gotten the jump on my brain? I would have walked out on a much-needed job with the essential benefits! When I did earn my position as a checker, it was with a new attitude and an understanding of how to be a team player. The job was a bit awkward at the beginning since I was the new kid fresh out of high school, and several co-workers felt it was necessary to take me under their wing to train and educate. Eventually, I did come to appreciate their good intentions, and it was invaluable for my growth and maturity.

I had turned twenty when, as mentioned earlier, my younger brother Tom started nagging me about meeting his friend Greg. At that time, Greg and I were both working full-time and were satisfied to live for the moment. Like most young adults, we were, enjoying the bar scene and coming and going as we pleased with no accountability other than to ourselves. During this stage of our lives, it would be accurate to say that we were in the process of constructing and defining our individuality, and we were comfortable living by our own rules.

Greg, who was an apprentice plumber and pipefitter, shared an apartment with his best friend Kevin, and I lived with my parents and six younger siblings while saving to move out. He was also an incredibly handsome, outgoing, and independent person who radiated self-confidence. I on the other hand was painfully shy, kind, dependable and responsible. I was also a hard worker and a master at hiding my insecurities behind a mask of confidence.

When Greg and I started dating, neither of us was looking for a serious commitment; we just wanted to enjoy each other's company without any expectations. Our dates entailed meeting up after work for a few drinks, going out for dinner, enjoying a movie or rides on his motorcycle, or hanging out at his apartment. Greg's routine was to party with friends on Friday night and ride the dirt trails on Saturday with Tom and other friends. When we were together, I did most of the conversing because he was a man of few words unless he had the insight to share, a joke to tell, or was in a playful or smartass mood. Within months of our relationship, we were together more than apart, and somehow, before I knew it, he had breached my protective barrier and became my best friend. I know it sounds hokey, but loving him was as natural as breathing, and for the first time, I had a relationship built on mutual respect, trust, and love. I will always be grateful to Tom for his hindsight that we would make a perfect couple and refusing to let me hide.

After a year of dating, we braved the subject of marriage and had an intense conversation about what our expectations were and the magnitude of a lifelong commitment to one another. By the end of the night, confident that we were ready to take this leap of faith, we became engaged. Our aspiration for matrimony was to attain a union comparable to those of our parents, who made it seem relatively easy.

On February 4, 1978, Greg and I courageously stood before our family and friends to exchange wedding vows. Greg, being raised Baptist, was less than excited about the long Catholic wedding of my faith, but he and his family endured the stand-up, sit down, and kneel of the ceremony. Cindy and Mike loaned us their car for the wedding so Greg could hide his prized green metallic Dodge Charger in a friend's garage to prevent from being decorated. Knowing that I am a huge Elvis fan, my thoughtful groom chose Memphis, Tennessee for our honeymoon destination so that I could see Graceland. We left behind a nasty Iowa snowstorm for the pleasantly warm weather of Tennessee and began our destiny of discovering, adapting, growing, and building a life together.

While we knew intellectually that married life would be an adjustment, like most newlyweds we were more excited and focused having a pleasurable adventure. The reality check was quite enlightening, though, as we endured some intense moments as we learned to share the same space, juggle routines, and accept and embrace each other's personality quirks. By the end of our first year of wedded bliss, we lost some of those polished manners that we had once used so diligently, and a disagreement turned into a yelling match. Several days passed with us scarcely speaking to one other, each night taking that anger to bed without either of us attempting to resolve the situation. When we finally stopped acting like spoiled children, we admitted that the thing that bothered us most was going to bed still angry and turning our backs to one another. We made a promise never again to go to bed without a kiss goodnight even if we were still irritated with one another. Making that pact was the first of countless life lessons that were invaluable and paramount for us building a resilient marriage. Another reality check, there is no such thing as "wedded bliss," at least not the way it is described in fairytales!

We learned to channel our bad moments into valuable relationship lessons and continued to grow from there. Upon reflection, I believe that God had a hand in giving us the capacity to learn these essential relationship skills to prepare us for what lay ahead in our lives. Thankfully, we evolved as a couple with the realization that empathy was a necessary element of our relationship, which ultimately became an essential component for us as parents. By choosing at the very beginning to make our marriage a priority, it fundamentally enabled us to build a strong foundation that we worked at consistently to make into a lasting relationship. Perseverance was only part of the strategy we utilized to endure the consistent hurdles. We also had to learn to compromise, acquire patience, offer apologies, and forgive faults. In my experience, it takes a great deal of love, faith, a deep commitment, respect, hard work, and a damn good sense of humor to build a solid foundation in any relationship.

After two years of marriage and countless questions about when we were having a baby, we finally contemplated becoming parents. As usual, we talked extensively over the pros and cons of our decision and conceded that creating a little human could be a blessing but also a disadvantage as well. Parenthood was an enormous responsibility that would entail a significant lifestyle change in that we could no longer pick up and go at our leisure. The financial strain to the budget was also a consideration, and if I heard it a hundred times, I heard it a thousand times growing up, it was not cheap or easy to raise kids. Greg was more apprehensive about being a parent, which was understandable since he lacked my experience of being an older sibling of six. Eventually we deemed ourselves mature enough, responsible enough, and dedicated enough to make a child a priority in our life. Once we made the decision, I quickly became pregnant and was ecstatic about finally fulfilling my childhood dream of being a mom!

Once the jubilation passed, though, I was fretting about the reality of being responsible for the life of our baby. After dreaming about having a child, I was now experiencing the surreal and frightening reality. If Greg had similar emotions, he never showed or expressed them. His reaction to the news of his impending fatherhood was merely an acceptance of the inevitable. Thank goodness, my pregnancy spared me the unpleasant symptom of morning sickness. That sensation of the first flutter was bizarre, and the tickle of movement was exciting, but neither of those was as impressive as that definite kick. The loss of my waistline meant that the baby was healthy and growing. As my pregnancy advanced, that alleged glow folks gush about faded, and my naïve enthusiasm vanished as my girth multiplied.

By the nine-month mark I had lost visual contact with my feet, and fatigue took root as my sense of humor turned into a menacing growl. My futile attempts at finding a comfortable position on our worn-out mattress became a nightly battle with me being the loser. The once simple procedure of shaving my legs now required some degree of acrobatics and an occasional band-aide. However, the final indignity was having to resort to that embarrassing "rocking motion" to stand. I was awkward and felt unattractive, and the teasing from my family regarding my size only validated my belief that I resembled a moving mountain. This element of pregnancy was not what I had envisioned in my dreams of impending motherhood. Another reality check!

On April 18, 1980, my exact due date, we headed to the hospital and three hours later, at 3:06 a.m., Stephanie was born. I was exhausted, but the inconvenience of pregnancy and pain of delivery were swiftly forgotten once I held our beautiful and healthy seven-pound daughter. Giving thanks to the Lord for our precious gift, I cradled her securely in my arms as I smoothed down her fine layer of black hair. While gazing into her murky blue eyes and admiring her adorable little chipmunk cheeks, it dawned on me that I was holding the legacy of mine and Greg's love. If my heart could feel such a profound love for my first child, how deeply was it for my parents, with nine of us? That was my first understanding of the statement that no one can truly appreciate their parents until they become one.

Being an older sister may have groomed me for this moment, but the enormity of the obligation that came with being a parent had just started to register. That feeling of tranquility was beginning to fade away, and in its place was an unvarnished truth that this little girl was now utterly defenseless and solely dependent on me and Greg. We may have felt competent, mature, and ready to have a child, but the impact of her arrival made us acutely aware of what novices we were in the role of parenting. Ready or not, the clock of accountability was ticking, and we had better succeed in this endeavor since it was our decision, not hers, to create her life. There was no other option than to become equipped and thrive at being committed, loving, nurturing, and attentive parents.

Stephanie was an adorable, happy, and cuddly baby for about four months, and then all hell broke loose. She developed colic and would shriek and stiffen her little body from the pain of not being able to expel gas. My attempts to comfort her were ineffective, and the doctor's reassurance that this stage would pass did little to ease my already frazzled nerves. The best method to calm her would entail long stroller rides around the neighborhood or car rides when the weather was terrible. As soon as she drifted off to sleep, I headed home, and Greg cautiously lifted our Sleeping Beauty, carriage and all, and brought her into the house. We held our breaths and prayed all would remain quiet, as he gently lowered the stroller or car seat to the floor as we tiptoed out of the room. There seemed to be more bad days than good as the ugly colic stage persistently undermined my confidence as a mom and pushed me toward the crazy zone.

The longer the crying spells dragged on, the more inadequate and depressed I felt. My attempts to fold Stephanie's little body in half to help relieve the gas did not bring comfort. Often her cries turned into screams, and then I was crying. Greg stood by helplessly watching as I tried to alleviate her pain, and when the misery was too much, he retreated to the garage to escape the wails of mother and child. His ability to hide in the garage pissed me off, and I resented the hell out of him. Did he even once consider that I wanted to do the same thing? Had we not created this screaming child together? Did my being a mom mean that I was the sole parent when things got difficult? When I hit him with my assumptions, he assured me he only left because there was nothing he could do for either of us to make it better and could not endure watching.

Parenting was more complicated than either of us had anticipated, and when it was too much for me, I took our crying daughter over to Mom who always seemed to be able to ease Stephanie's pain. She used the same techniques that had failed me, and that only made me feel more inadequate. When I shared my feelings with Mom, she explained that I was unable to calm Stephanie because my stress was making the situation worse. Naturally, I instantly became defensive thinking she was placing the blame on me, but Mom was trying to clarify that I needed to be less tense. Yeah, like that was an easy solution living with a colicky baby! Then, just as the doctor predicted, the colic was gone, and she was again our happy little girl.

Stephanie grew quickly, and her teetering steps turned into a confident walk, and babbling noises became words and sentences. Her contagious giggle complimented her sweet disposition, and she had such an inquisitive nature, which certainly enhanced her ability to watch, listen, and learn. Her hair faded from black to light blonde, then almost to white, and the ringlets that encircled her head bounced in unison with her step. She was such a tender heart, and just a stern "NO" would make her bottom lip quiver and her eyes fill with tears. She was healthy, happy, loving, obedient, compassionate, and vivacious. Stephanie truthfully was the type of child parents dream of raising and we shined because she made it so darn easy. Our lives seemed picture perfect, and under the illusion that we had a handle on this parenting thing, we decided when Stephanie turned three that perhaps she needed a sibling.

Well, if you have been reading without skimming, you already know how that decision turned out! All joking aside, my attempt to get pregnant a second time took longer than it did with Stephanie. When I finally did get pregnant, it happened just as we lost Greg's dad in a horrific car accident, which caused difficulties in the early stages of the pregnancy. Since Rebecca's birth, the journey may have been turbulent and with hardships, but it has been a privilege and a blessing to be her mom. The adventure has been life-changing, but one of the purest gifts from individuals with special needs is that their love sincerely comes from their heart. For them, life is seen through the eyes of a child, which helps them to not dwell on issues, and they recover quickly from upsets, which enables them to look instead for the fun. We could all definitely learn from their ability to live in the moment, but instead, we all too often let our intellect be in the driver's seat and overload our minds and hearts.

I blossomed into the individual I am today by the grace of God, because He chose me to be given the gift of Rebecca. Her many struggles brought extraordinary people into my life who encouraged me and ultimately made me a better mom. They imparted wisdom and techniques which facilitated my ability to cultivate the necessary skills for successfully raising a special needs individual. Greg and I faced unique challenges with our parenting skills because we had to parent Rebecca differently than Stephanie. The parent playbook that we developed while raising Stephanie was relatively worthless where Rebecca was concerned. We may have been parents for a second time, but we were novices at how to raise a child with special needs.

We had decided before Stephanie was born that we were committed to being solely responsible for raising her and that meant I would be a stay at home mom and Greg would continue providing for our family's financial needs. His job did not have sick days so if he did not work there was no pay for the day and that was the reason he was not able to join me when I got the painful diagnoses of Rebecca's disabilities. Since I could not call him at work, I had to wait for him to get home to relay the results of the tests, which gave me most of the day to process the shock before I had to tell him. After I finished explaining the diagnoses, he just sat there staring down at the floor trying to digest the difficult news. When he finally looked up at me, the extreme sadness in his eyes probably mirrored my own when I was told of the results. He took a deep breath and then told me that he trusted me to take care of whatever came next and just like that, I was put in the driver's seat. He was confident that I was the more capable parent and therefore the best candidate for the job.

My frenzied objections, namely that I did not have a clue how to deal with this disorder or have the tools to undertake such a huge endeavor, did not sway him in the least. He had made the decision that I was to be the primary advocate for Rebecca and then pointed out, quite painfully, that I was the non-working parent and that it was logical for me to take the lead. His focus was to work diligently to pay the additional expenses that were incurred and then fade into the background, only coming forward when needed or forced. Avoidance became his method of distancing himself from our new reality of Rebecca's diagnoses and a comfortable position for most of the journey. When he alone decided that I would be the parent to step up, care for, and fight for our daughter, it initiated a shift in our relationship. It triggered a fracture in what had always been a strong parenting partnership and left me feeling unsupported.

In Greg's defense, he was only operating from the false persona that I presented to him, as well as to others, that I could handle most anything that came my way. Years of practice had made me a master at sufficiently hiding behind my protective mask and giving everyone the impression that I was tough when really, I had my share of insecurities and then some. Now all those years of pretending had put me in this predicament and forced me to be honest with Greg. I had kept my secret for so long that it took extreme courage to be that exposed and vulnerable in sharing my personal and tormenting deficits. I was an emotionally weak person with a severe lack of self-confidence, but my pretend façade had so thoroughly convinced Greg that my confession failed to sway him. Coming clean made no difference, and he remained firm that I was more capable of addressing Rebecca's particular needs. It was then that I realized I had missed my calling and should have studied acting! This situation was a turning point for me and made me reach beyond my insecurities and find the resolution to tackle this problem.

No matter how upsetting they may have seemed at the time, none of my prior experiences carried such dire consequences as the prospect of failing Rebecca. Her welfare came first, and that pushed me to focus on finding people that could help. Since I was the first sibling to have a child with disabilities, my family was as perplexed as I was on where to start, and yet oddly enough, they all believed that I could handle this situation. Perhaps my belief that I had missed my calling as an actor was not so farfetched. Life had shoved me out from behind the curtain, and although I did not have a script, being in the spotlight gave me the courage to believe that I could play the part I was given.

As mentioned earlier, while parenting Rebecca, Greg and I had to devise different strategies from those we used with Stephanie. We also made a pact to stay united when dealing with the girls, and if we disagreed with something the other had implemented, it was to be discussed in private. There was a consistent dynamic in our partnership with me being the warden and Greg, the enforcer who stepped in when the girls did not follow my direction. They always tried to become smaller when their dad became part of the conversation. They did not like when he looked over his glasses, snapped his fingers, pointed the finger at them, or thundered. Occasionally, I did get soft when they cried, but Greg was always immune to the tears. The girls loved cuddling with their dad when he came home for work and I was preparing dinner. I tried to capture those sweet moments in pictures as much as possible. The years passed, and so did the cuddling, which transitioned into the attack and wrestling phase, of which one of my delicate knickknacks became the occasional casualty.

My journey in finding effective ways of dealing with Rebecca's ADHD brought another division for Greg and myself. He was more open to using the medication, but I could not accept the consequences that came with a prescription. I am thankful that Greg supported my desire to implement the K-P Diet because we were once again a team. Sometimes I do wonder what would have happened to Rebecca if I had surrendered to the pressure to medicate her. I honestly doubt she would be as successful as she is today, especially since parents, their children, teachers, and caregivers are still struggling with disruptive behaviors of ADHD, even with the use of medication. It is astounding to me that even after thirty years the medical community's number one "solution" is to medicate these children when there is evidence out there that the same or better results can be achieved with diet and behavior modification, at least in many cases.

Greg has shared with me that if he had been in charge of Rebecca's care, he doubts that things would have turned out as well as they have for her. He sincerely believed that medication was the most straightforward choice to solve our problems and amazed at my determination and ability to devour so many books to educate myself. Most likely, if I had not set out to get a better understanding of Rebecca's disorder, I too might have accepted medication as the answer. As far as her successes, it took a tribe of family, friends, teachers, and strangers to get Rebecca to this place in her life. The road toward Rebecca's independence took her a bit longer than expected, but she is happy and more confident in her abilities than ever.

Life is different when you finally reach that long-awaited "empty nester" phase and discover how much you have changed. You look at the gray hair, wrinkles, groans of movement, and bellies protruding from abundance and wonder where all the years went. We began this adventure, young, frisky, and agile youngsters full of love and aspirations for a grand life and what we received was incredible, aggravating, joyful, painful, and an abundance of blessings. There are two beautiful young women and a grandson to show for our love, and in my opinion that is something to be very proud of. I truthfully cannot think of a better journey than one with your best friend, for better or worse, as you take on life with a heart full of love, faith that a higher power is watching over you, and the courage to hold steady when the winds of life come howling through.

Greg and I can sit for hours utterly comfortable in our silence, look at one another, and feel confident that we made the best decision forty-one years ago when we took that leap of faith. To be able to build and sustain a relationship that has lasted this long is one hell of an accomplishment in this current "throw away" world where all too often people and relationships are expendable. I still chuckle about those doubters who thought when Greg and I tied the knot that we would not make it this long because of our differences. He takes his time to decide and needs to be sure that he has all the facts, and I sometimes jump before I am sure of the outcome only to have it bite me in the ass later. He is slow to anger, and I embrace the Irish gene but thankfully have developed a longer fuse over the years. Greg believes that I can fight my own battles and expects me to be victorious while I see myself more like a warrior out of necessity. In my heart, I still cling to the vision of him as my knight in shining armor and protector. We balance one another out, and I guess that comes from our life experience and always trusting that we have each other's backs.

It makes my heart heavy for those who go into marriage wanting that lifelong adventure, only to be kicked in the teeth by losing a loved one in death or by someone who does not have the same vision. Our sweet Stephanie is just such a casualty of trusting someone with her heart, who sadly failed to have the same beliefs and desires for marriage. The blessing from her heartache is Chayton, our grandson. Stephanie makes us proud and is doing such a fantastic job of raising her son as a single parent and "Little Man," as I call him, is a miniature of his momma. Chayton is a sponge, watching, listening, and learning from what is going on around him and just as eager to grow up. I hear myself telling him, as I did to his momma, to slow down and enjoy being a kid because being an adult is more an illusion of fun than it is.

Would I retake this journey knowing all that I do now? Yes - in a heartbeat! - because I have learned so much, achieved more than I thought I could, and discovered that my purpose is to share my story. The journey had many twists, turns, and challenges, but it helped me to grow, brought individuals into my life to instruct me, guide me, support me, and ultimately inspire me. They were the lifeline I searched for, and they had a hand in making me stronger so that I can now be your beacon of light. None of us has to be alone in dealing with our child's disabilities, and I have blazed a trail for you between the pages of this book with a safe means to manage your child's ADHD, and possibly other disorders, with lifestyle changes.

In Closing

My story is more than an insight about how I safely raised an ADHD child, but also about developing determination and endurance while enduring the hard knocks life sometimes deals us. Life does not give us a break from other situations because we are busy dealing with something else. During this emotional and sometimes painful process, I learned to trust my instincts, believe in myself, develop resiliency, and most importantly, cultivated the woman I am today. The outcome from my journey is not only about Rebecca's successes, but my personal growth too, and an intense desire to help other parents like myself. From my story, may you find hope, encouragement, and be uplifted as you travel the frustrating and challenging road of raising an ADHD child. Today, there is an abundance of help available for you, and the first step in anything is to have faith and courage.

If you found something of value or have any questions, please feel free to email me at shirlcsmith@gmail.com or visit my Facebook Author Page at http://www.facebook.com/Shirl Crimmins Smith. I also have a quick read book on Amazon to give you additional insight into my perspectives and my journey. http://www.amazon.com/-/e/B07SFZ1R8J ab

About the Author

Shirl Crimmins Smith has over thirty years' experience and knowledge that she utilized to develop techniques that enriched the health and education of her daughter with ADHD, Learning Disabilities, and Minimal Brain Disorder. It was from the trenches of her daily battle with the chaotic and hostile behavior of then-four-year-old Rebecca that she vowed to search for answers.

She had depleted her arsenal of parenting tricks with her obstinate daughter and headed to her local library simply looking for clarification and strategies for dealing with the ADHD symptoms. However, what she discovered was that trying to decipher the information was like falling into a deep rabbit hole. The multidimensional disorder was complex and understanding it would entail reading over 110 books, multiple articles, and watching numerous televised programs. Eventually, Shirl's determination to find a safe and effective method for managing the behaviors of ADHD led her to Dr. Ben F. Feingold's, *Why Your Child Is Hyperactive*. This book changed the way Shirl viewed the disorder and one she credits in her daughter's success today.

Smith followed the all-natural diet and strategies from Dr. Feingold's book which achieved extraordinary improvements regarding Rebecca's erratic behaviors. The change was so dramatic that word reached the local newspaper who sent a reporter to the house for an interview. Both mother and child were featured in the front-page article, along with their photo, explaining her success with the Feingold Diet. Shirl also attributes much of her success in raising Rebecca to the strategies she cultivated over the seventeen years she worked with school psychologists, speech and language specialists, social workers, and Special Education teachers.

Over the years, Shirl has helped multiple parents in giving them a better understanding of ADHD, an explanation of how to use the Feingold diet, and offering productive parenting strategies. She is always willing to share her time and expertise with parents searching for an alternative to the use of medication to help manage their child's ADHD at home and in school. She has also been asked to create a special cookbook for busy parents with ADHD children.

http://www.facebook.com/ShirlCrimminsSmith
http://www.amazon.com/-/e/B07SFZ1R8J
www.ShirlCrimminsSmith.com